HANDBOOK OF BIOSTATISTICS

A Review and Text

HANDBOOK OF BIOSTATISTICS

A Review and Text

Christos P. Carvounis MD, MACP, FCCP, FACN

Professor of Medicine
at the State University of New York at Stony Brook

and
Chief of the Division of Nephrology
at the Nassau County Medical Center

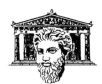

The Parthenon Publishing Group
International Publishers in Medicine, Science & Technology

NEW YORK   LONDON

Published in the USA by
The Parthenon Publishing Group Inc.
One Blue Hill Plaza
PO Box 1564, Pearl River,
New York 10965, USA

Published in the UK and Europe by
The Parthenon Publishing Group Limited
Casterton Hall, Carnforth,
Lancs., LA6 2LA, UK

Library of Congress Cataloging-in-Publication Data

Carvounis, Christos P.
  Handbook of biostatistics: a review and text/Christos P.
Carvounis
    p. cm.
    Includes index
    ISBN 1-85070-749-9
    1. Biometry – Handbooks, manuals, etc.   2. Biometry – Examinations,
questions, etc. – Handbooks, manuals, etc.   I. Title.
    [DNLM: 1 Biometry.   2. Biometry examination questions.   WA950
C331h 1998]
RA409.C325   1998
570'.1'5195 – dc21
DNLM/DLC
for Library of Congress   98-44804
                                                                      CIP

British Library Cataloguing in Publication Data

Carvounis, C. P.
  Handbook of biomedical statistics: a review and text
  1. Medical statistics – Handbooks, manuals, etc. 2. Biometry
  I. Title
  610.2'1

ISBN 1-85070-749-9

Typeset by H&H Graphics, Blackburn, UK
Printed and bound by Bookcraft (Bath) Ltd., Midsomer Norton, UK

To Georgia,
my wife and best friend,
for being passionate yet patient,
flexible yet straightforward,
for being herself!

Contents

PREFACE

Why yet another textbook of Biostatistics? There is little question that a substantial number of well-written textbooks exist. However the vast majority belong to one of the following categories. Either too long and technical or too short and superficial. This often leaves the average physician, medical student or biology worker dissatisfied. He or she needs answers to questions about the statistical analysis needed to deal with a specific clinical or basic research project or the appropriate selection of statisical analysis in a given paper. (S)he needs a reasonably brief, yet deep enough treatise that will explain the specific statistical analysis needed, without going into extreme technical detail. This is of utmost importance since the validity of any biological research depends on the relevance and significance of the questions addressed and the methods used to address these questions. Statistics represent the centerpiece for any methodology. Consider, for instance, if one fails to demonstrate the impact of a new therapy for a given disease because of lack of understanding of statistics (lack of control, fewer subjects than needed, or inappropriate statistical analysis). In a sense this represents a major disfavor to humanity! (not to mention the time and expense incurred). On the other hand the careless suggestion of a difference when in reality no such difference is present, for instance, if subjects are not randomized correctly, can lead to equally deleterious effects.

The other issue often encountered is that, for the most part, the authors of statistical books are professional biostatisticians who often do not appreciate the background or specific needs of the biology worker. After spending a significant amount of my time helping my colleagues to prepare their grants or scientific papers, I obtained a different perspective of their needs. Furthermore, I gave many courses on Biostatistics for postgraduate groups in my own Institution as well as others. This experience allowed me a clearer understanding of their difficulties and requirements. This textbook, therefore, was produced having all these objectives in mind. It represents an extensive revised form of the handouts I used for the courses. I have placed special emphasis on including all frequently used techniques. In particular, I have made sure that after reading this textbook, one could select the appropriate statistical method, once the initial steps (collection of data, randomisation of subjects into control and experimental groups, and determination of the number of subjects to participate in the study) have been dealt with. A conscious effort was put into presenting the different analytical methods as part of one system with a similar underlying syllogism. Student's *t* test and analysis of variance are presented as extensions of each other, rather than conceptually separate techniques. Similarly, linear regression and analysis of nominal data (chi-square and comparison of survival curves) are also discussed collectively as techniques exploring the variation of data points from the mean (sum of squares).

In addition to the topics covered traditionally in texts of biostatistics and epidemiology, I have made sure that more modern significant trends were also included. Evidence-based medicine has become a major player in the education of medical students in the last 5 years. The modern physician is expected to be able to transform probabilities into ratio, compute the likelihood that a given is present, and be exact about his/her expectations regarding the effects of a given therapeutic regimen. Extensive discussion with examples in Chapters 2 and 3 deal with the interrelations of probability to odds ratio, the use of likelihood ratio and its optical counterpart, the receiver operated curve. Special emphasis is placed on the significance of a receiver operated curve, and the ability to identify the best cutoff point for a diagnostic test. In Chapter 7, a detailed discussion explains how one can use ratio and possibilities of therapeutic regimens to allow one to identify, in real terms, these issues. Appropriate use of such technique permits meaningful conclusions to questions such as how many people will it take to treat with a given drug or surgical procedure so as to prevent a death or to normalize a given pathologic finding.

Each chapter includes examples with step-by-step analysis of the solutions of the different situations encountered. At the end of the chapter a brief synopsis of the most pertinent points is offered. A variety of questions and answers are provided to permit a better understanding of the different topics. Finally, a number of appendices are offered to evaluate significance with the different statistical techniques.

It is only fair to conclude by expressing my gratitude to the many individuals who gave me significant help to bring this book to its present form. I would like to thank Drs Laurie Ward and Donald Feinfeld for their encouragement and their most useful suggestions. I appreciate the support of Dr Noel Meltzer throughout the writing of this book. I thank Mrs Marie Murphy for her excellent secretarial support. Finally I would like express my appreciation to Mrs Christina Esposito for her assistance in making the figures that accompany the text. This book would never have been completed without their support.

CHAPTER 1

Introduction

WHY SHOULD WE LEARN STATISTICS?

Statistics is the science that allows us to formulate and describe complex data in a short form, easily understood by all professionals. It allows us to compare data and gives us probabilities of the likelihood of events. The first component of statistics is the presentation of data and is called **descriptive statistics.** The second component, that of comparing data or identifying probabilities, is called **inferential statistics.**

A few examples will permit some insight into the significance of statistics in our scientific life. Let us assume that we have the hematocrits of all members of a group, say that of the 106 students in the 8th grade of a given school. It will be rather cumbersome to present all data points, and even then, one may still have a difficult time drawing meaningful conclusions. By contrast, the same data could be presented as 40 ± 2 and if one knows **the language of statistics** (i.e. the meaning of mean and standard deviation) a more comprehensive understanding of the characteristic (hematocrit) in a given population (8th graders in that school) will emerge. However, there may be more than one way to present the data. Let us suppose that a hematocrit of 37 is considered the cut off below which a subject is called anemic. If 5 out of 100 children had a hematocrit below 37, one may present the same data as 95% of the children were normal and 5% were anemic. There are specific rules within **descriptive statistics** that tell us which way is appropriate or even acceptable and which is unacceptable or misleading. It is imperative therefore, to learn the statistical language and its rules if you are to be able to comprehend (either in reading scientific literature or in producing it), just as you need to learn any language correctly if you are to use it to communicate. Now let us assume that you would like to compare the hematocrits mentioned above with the hematocrits of another group of 8th grade students from another school in a different school district, state or even country with different socioeconomic, cultural or nutritional backgrounds. It is obvious that you will encounter several problems. It becomes very difficult to examine all the members of the relevant population, so you may have to resort to representative samples. It is, therefore, critical that the selection be **random,** precluding bias. Random selection implies that all individuals of the population have an equal chance of being selected. Otherwise major bias may be present. For instance, if you sample only students attending a given sporting event, you may inadvertently concentrate mostly on boys. Similarly, if you sample students from the class basketball team, your observations may be skewed toward the more physically fit students and may not be a representative sample of the class as a whole. Another issue is the selection of an **appropriate size** of a sample so that you will be able to find differences if they exist, or to avoid describing differences, if indeed they are not present. Finally, one has to select an **appropriate statistical method** to perform a comparison. All these are issues dealt with in **inferential statistics.**

Keep in mind that we all do statistics daily, except that we do it instinctively, emotionally and unscientifically, and we often draw the wrong conclusions. For example, when we are about to buy a new home we ask questions such as: Is the construction good? Would this structure require minimal repair in the next ten years? Is the price logical? Will the resale price be significant? For that, we or experts that we hire for that purpose, compare the data of the house under consideration with similar houses they have encountered, and draw conclusions accordingly. If our experience is small or skewed, it could lead to the wrong answers. There are similar situations in the everyday practice of medicine. It is our experience and reading that suggest that a 50-year-old man with chest pain and diaphoresis has a high likelihood of myocardial infarction and we admit him to the coronary care unit. By contrast, chest pain and sweating in a 13-year-old child participating in a contact sport suggest a different etiology.

Statistics are predominantly needed in more **probabilistic** and **less predictive** sciences such as medicine (Figure 1). In a predictive science such as physics, to find out how fast a 300 g stone will reach the ground if dropped from a height of 30 yards, one has only to only apply the data in the appropriate formula to obtain an accurate answer. In art, on the other hand, the evaluation of a given piece depends to a great extent on subjective criteria. For instance, there have been heated debates on whether the Eiffel Tower in Paris is one of the world's most wonderful structures or an architectural disaster. Medicine falls somewhere in between. There are numerous and complex physical/chemical events occurring simultaneously which cannot be evaluated separately.

For instance, if one wants to determine the time of induction, or return, of a given reflex, say that of the achilles tendon, the issue is more complicated than it appears initially. In this case we are dealing with

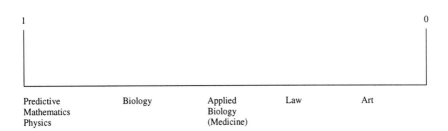

| 1 | | | | 0 |

Predictive	Biology	Applied	Law	Art
Mathematics		Biology		
Physics		(Medicine)		

Figure 1 Subjects are divided according to their predictability (1 represents high predictability, 0 represents low predictability). Statistics, are particularly useful for subjects that contain a lot of definite information, but quite complex, thus with a high level of insecurity. These subjects will be found in the middle of this scale. Biology, and applied biology (medicine) represent a classical example where statistics will be of great significance. The statistics used to deal with such issues are called **biostatistics**

transmission of electrical potential difference across many nerves and transmission to muscles, making relevant calculations more tedious and the specific data less well known. Furthermore, the specific functions are affected by several other components of our internal milieu such as the level of thyroid hormones. To complicate matters, this will represent just one out of many concommitant functions of a total inhomogenous system, our body. It is, therefore, easy to appreciate why biological sciences in general, and applied biology such as medicine, in particular, are probabilistic in nature. As a result, a good grasp of statistics is essential for one to be effective in this field.

WHY LEARN STATISTICS OURSELVES INSTEAD OF CONSULTING EXPERTS?

One important reason is that it is not always possible to have professional help available when the need arises, since there are few statisticians and we often need statistical evaluations. For example, imagine reading the medical literature. If you are to accept the findings and conclusions of a given paper it implies that you accept the methodology, and in particular, that the statistical methods are correct. It is obvious that inappropriate statistics will cast doubt on the conclusions suggested by the authors. This is not an insignificant problem found only in small journals. When a number of papers from 30 well known journals, including the *New England Journal of Medicine* and *Annals of Internal Medicine*, were evaluated, it was found that 80% had statistical errors! Even though increased emphasis has recently been placed on statistics by the editors, it is easy to recognize why it is important to have a good grasp of statistics oneself! This is not to imply that advice from experts should not be sought if one plans an original study or needs help in the formulation or comparison of complex data.

WHY NOT USE A COMPUTER STATISTICS PROGRAM INSTEAD OF LEARNING STATISTICS?

To use a statistical program implies that at the very least you have already selected the appropriate method. In other words, that you already know about statistics. Furthermore, it is important to realize that the computer will not help you in collecting your data, avoiding bias, or selecting the most appropriate way to formulate or compare data. Also, the computer will do nothing for you when you attempt to find out whether a given paper used appropriate statistics and whether its conclusions are valid and believable. In short, the computer can help you with calculations, but it is imperative that you have a grasp of the basic concepts.

HOW MANY CATEGORIES OF DATA ARE THERE AND WHY IS IT IMPORTANT TO KNOW THESE CATEGORIES?

As mentioned above, the hematocrit can be presented quantitatively by using a continuous scale; it is then called **continuous** data. In continuous data there are infinite possible numbers between two points. For example, if we deal with 100 and 101, one could also consider that in between them we could find 100.4, 100.58, 100.6967 and so on. The second characteristic is that in continuous data the scale is homogeneous so that a distance 'X' is identical at any position on the scale. In simple terms the difference in weight between 101 and 100 or 165 and 164 is the same. Continuous data could be further subdivided into **interval** and **ratio** scales. The only difference between them is that in an *interval* scale the zero point is arbitrarily defined and does not indicate the total absence of the property determined. This is in contrast to a ratio scale in which zero indeed suggests absence of the property. For instance temperature expressed in degrees Fahrenheit or Celsius is an example of an interval scale. In contrast, weight determination in kg, time in seconds, and heart rate in beats per minute all represent examples of ratio scales. With regard to statistical analysis (presentation or comparisons), this division is of no significance and all such data could be considered collectively as **continuous** data.

Data may be expressed also in a qualitative way. **Ordinal data** is where data are ranked and presented in the form: first, second . . . tenth. The average in such a presentation is the score of the average performer (**median**) as opposed to an average of the different data (**mean**). In this form of presentation variation is presented either as the range or as quartiles rather than variance, standard deviation, or standard error of the mean, as is often the case with continuous data.

Use of ordinal data is suggested when either the data are semiquantitative or when there are outliers (and the data are skewed). By semiquantitative we mean data where the difference between two points is not precisely determined on a continuous scale. For instance, NY Heart Association classes of heart failure, or the stages of tumors such as Dukes class II and so forth represent such examples. Please note that while a cardiac patient with class I disease is doing better than the patient with class II, who in turn is better off than the patient with class III, one has no right to say that the difference between the first and the second patient is the same as the one between the second and the third patient. In other words, classes I, II, and III allow ranking but not precise evaluations (semiquantitative data). Even though the scoring appears continuous, there is no consistent degree of difference among rank.

As already stated, another use of ordinal data is when the data in a continuous scale contains outliers, that is, data points far away from the mean and the bulk of the observations. In such cases, one should *not* use continuous data because that could be both erroneous and misleading. Think, for example, of examining the salaries of senior faculty members and administrators in a hospital. To make matters simple, a sample of four is selected from each group. Each of the physician salaries is $100 000. Three of the administrator salaries were $50 000 and one, that of the CEO is $250 000 (i.e. 50 000, 50 000, 50 000, 250 000 dollars). If one treats these data as continuous then the conclusion is that there is no difference between the groups since the mean salary of each group is $100 000. A better way to deal with the data is to say that the average (median) physician draws $100 000 while the average (median) administrator draws $50 000. As we will discuss in Chapter 2, use of continuous data (mean) is allowed only when the data are normally distributed. In the presence of outliers, and thus skewed data, ordinal data is preferable.

Another way to express data is qualitatively, whereby data are identified as members of a category and are known as *nominal* data. For instance, the hematocrit of people could be expressed as normal versus anemic, weight as normal versus obese, and so forth. It is understood that some characteristics can only be expressed as one of a few categories and such data should indeed be presented as nominal data. For example, in response to a treatment for cancer in a five-year period, one could belong to the group of either survivors or deceased. Similarly, one could be a man or a woman, have brown eyes or blue eyes, or have type A, B, AB or O blood. In all these examples, a subject belongs exclusively to one category by well-understood objective criteria. Furthermore, these categories do not allow for any further quantification, i.e. one cannot be more or less a survivor or dead, a man or a woman, type A or B.

The case, however, is very different when it comes to subjective subdivisions. Take the expression of body weight as normal or obese. Even though we have identified specific weights for any height to separate normalcy from obesity, it should be understood that this reflects the current weight standards which are often a reflection of culture and fashion. A visit to the Metropolitan Museum in New York and review of paintings of different eras and cultures should convince you that there have been times when what we presently call normal and obese were felt to be thin and normal, respectively. Thus, the first disadvantage of nominal data is that of subjectivity when the discrimination among groups reflects personal preference or epidemiologic criteria rather than physiologically distinct and relevant differences. However, a more important problem with nominal data is the fact that the data are clumped together, thus decreasing the discriminatory ability among groups. For example, think about the hematocrits of a sample of five from two groups of women. The data from group A are 37, 37, 38, 39, 41 and that of group B are 42, 43, 43, 44, 45. Using continuous data, one could express the hematocrits as 38.4 ± 1.7 and 43.4 ± 1.1 respectively, allowing one to say that the two groups differ with regard to their hematocrit, something that we will formally address later when considering inferential statistics. Alternatively, one could present the same data using nominal statistics if one assumes that normal hematocrit for women is above 36. In this case, the data of either group could be expressed as 100% normal. Implicit in this statement is that there is no difference between the groups, an obvious inaccuracy! In simple terms, it is imperative that we present data in its more robust[1] form if possible, i.e. continuous over ordinal and ordinal over nominal. There are only three situations where data may be appropriately expressed in nominal as opposed to continuous data. They are:

(a) **data belong to only one of a few categories**. For instance, one is either alive or dead, either a man or a woman. There is no meaningful category such as less alive or more dead. Thus there is a clear distinction between the *categories without intermediate values* (that prevent quantitative treatment);

(b) **the distinction into categories is physiologically valid.** For example, the population of adults could be divided into adults and elderly (i.e. over the age of 65 years). Although the distinction is somewhat artificial, it allows one to evaluate the biological behavior of a group with some common characteristics (for the most part they do not work, they live on pensions that are often less than salaries, they demonstrate progressive biologic deficits, etc);

---

[1]By more robust we define a technique that allows a more complete use of data. Obviously using the most 'robust' one will allow you to demonstrate differences among groups easier – when such differences exist

(c) **the results are similar by using either continuous or nominal data and distinction into categories (nominal) is done for simplicity and is physiologically acceptable.** For example, one may subdivide a population into those with good urinary concentration ability and those with concentration deficits, depending on whether their urine osmolality is higher or lower than 400 mosm/kg when given vasopressin or faced with stress (presumed high endogenous vasopressin). We recently found that patients admitted to the medical intensive care unit who have concentration deficit on admission have a markedly increased likelihood of developing either acute renal failure or dying during the admission. Dividing the data into two categories did not diminish the predictability of the model (as opposed to presenting Uosm as continuous data in a scale from 50–1200 mosm/kg) and allowed for a single and valid conclusion (i.e. concentrating defects predict ARF and mortality). We therefore elected to present the data in the form of two categories.

The *major necessity of categorizing data* into continuous, ordinal and nominal is that this *dictates the type of statistical technique that will be required* (Table 1). It is only after this step is complete that one may then start thinking about using a computer program. As shown in Table 1, we are looking at two types of data. One is the data of our immediate interest, the outcome of the study, often called the dependent variable. The type of input that operates on the outcome is called the independent variable. In order to understand these issues that at first appear confusing, let us consider two examples.

24-h urine creatinine equals the 24 h creatinine production and in turn reflects the size of our somatic proteins (muscle). Now let us assume you would like to compare two groups of patients (say diseased versus control) regarding their somatic protein. For that you elected 24-h urine creatinine as a measure of somatic protein. In this case, 24-h urine creatinine represents the outcome or dependent variable and is continuous data. The input or independent variable is the two different groups (diseased versus control) and is nominal data (bivariable). Going to Table 1 one finds that the appropriate test is Student's *t*-test. If more than two groups were to be evaluated (multivariable input), analysis of variance would have been the appropriate test. If the creatinine data contained outliers then the outcome should have been dealt in terms of ordinal data. Thus a Mann–Whitney U test and a Kruskall–Wallis would have been the appropriate selections for two or more groups.

Let us look at another example where you would like to evaluate the effects of a weight loss diet on somatic protein. In this case the outcome will also be 24-h urine creatinine (continuous) and the input two groups (control versus diet) nominal. However, in this example the two groups are composed of the same subjects before (control) and after dieting

Table 1 Method of finding the appropriate statistical test to use with the appropriate data

Input – Independent variables	Outcome (Dependent variables)					
	A. Continuous		*B. Ordinal*		*C. Nominal*	
	Unmatched	*Matched*	*Unmatched*	*Matched*	*Unmatched*	*Matched*
Nominal						
Invariable	Student-*t*	–	Wilcoxon signed rank test	–	Binomial (common events) Poisson (rare events)	
Variable	Student-*t* –	Student-*t* (paired)	Mann-Whitney U	Wilcoxin-signed rank test	Chi-square Fisher's exact Mantel–Haenszel	McNemar
Multivariable	One way analysis of variance (ANOVA)	Repeated Measures ANOVA	Kruskall-Wallis	Friedman	Log-rank Chi-square Mantel–Haenszel	Cochran Q
Continuous or Ordinal	– Linear regression – Multiple regression – Multiple correlation – Analysis of covariance (ANCOVA)		– Spearman correlation – Kendal tau – Kendal W		– Cox regression – Logistic regression – Discriminant analysis	

and are therefore considered to be 'matched'. In such a case, each subject represents his/her own control. You would then select the paired Student *t*-test for this study. If the study extends to include a recovery phase, (control, diet, post-diet) then a repeated measure ANOVA, is needed because the input is no longer bivariable but is multivariable. If the data contain outliers, ordinal data would be more appropriate and a Wilcoxon-signed rank test for two groups or a Kruskall–Wallis test for more than two groups are the indicated statistical methods.

Now let us move to yet another study where you would like to evaluate the accuracy of 24-h urine creatinine to predict somatic mass. In order to do that you take an established technique for determining somatic muscle, such as mid-arm muscle circumference (MAMC) expressed in cm. Every subject has measurement of MAMC and 24-h urine creatinine taken simultaneously. The 24-h creatinines are the data of interest or the outcome, (dependent variable) and are continuous data. The input in our example is MAMC, also continuous data. Thus the appropriate test to use is linear regression for a normal distribution of both MAMC and creatinine data. If one encounters outliers, then Spearman's correlation is the appropriate test.

TAKE HOME MESSAGES

- Identify the category to which data belong from your study or from the literature.
- Use the more feasible robust category which, in descending order is: continuous > ordinal > nominal;

    ordinal data: a) presence of outliers;
                                   b) semiquantitative;

    nominal data: a) outcome lacks grading (e.g. death, gender)
                                   b) physiologically meaningful and results not dissimilar from continuous;
- Identify separately categories of outcome (dependent variable) and input (independent variable) and select appropriate statistical method (Table 1).

QUESTIONS

What statistical method will you select if you plan to:
1. Evaluate the effect of a drug on cardiac output?
2. Evaluate the action of two or more drugs on cardiac output?
3. Compare the relationship of the 24-hour urine creatinine to mid-arm circumference?
4. Evaluate whether type A blood occurs more often in one ethnic group as opposed to another?

CHAPTER 2

Data distribution and probabilities – the heart of statistics and epidemiology

CONTINUOUS DATA

We have already mentioned that a primary aim of statistics is to tabulate data and to summarize them in a way that allows one to appreciate an average and the way the data are distributed around it. If we know that the average height of a 12-year-old girl is 155 cm, this will permit a comparison of a given girl of that age group to the height generally expected. Thus a girl with a height of 147 cm belongs to a rather short category and one with a height of 167 cm could be labeled as tall. Furthermore, if we are told that the bulk of such girls (95% or 99%) have a height between 140 and 170 cm, one may draw useful conclusions. A girl with a height of 128 cm would be seriously considered very different from the expected, and evaluation for a metabolic disorder would be in order. Similarly, a classmate with a height of 182 cm could be considered for evaluation for gigantism.

The first characteristic of any data is that of the central tendency and three different ones are used. The **mean** is, in a sense, the numerical average. The **median** is the value that divides the data into two sets, i.e. the number of data points above the median equals the number of data points below. The **mode** is the most frequently occurring number. In the case of normal distribution of data, the average (mean) divides the data equally (median) and also represents the most frequent data value (mode). If the values are different, then the data are skewed (non-normal distribution, see below).

While the determination of average (mean) is rather obvious (sum of observations divided by number of observations), the description of the dispersion of the data around the mean is more complex. A reasonable way to deal with that is to find the distance of every single observation (X_i) from the mean ($\bar{x}$) and identify the average variability (X_i minus $\bar{x}$). One obvious way of doing this would be to sum up all variabilities and divide them by the number of observations. However, this will not work,

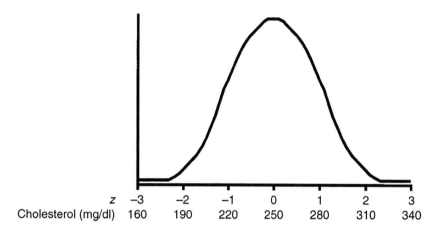

z	−3	−2	−1	0	1	2	3
Cholesterol (mg/dl)	160	190	220	250	280	310	340

Figure 2 A normal distrbution curve showing mean frequency distribution of a normally distributed population

since by definition, the positive difference data (data higher than the mean) will equal the negative data (data lower than the mean) and their sum will equal 0. In order to eliminate the sign one could square the differences and then sum them (sum of the squares) and divide them by the number of observations. This parameter is called **variance** and is an important one (we will use it later in the so-called analysis of variance). In actuality, instead of dividing by the number of observations, n, we actually divide by n – 1[1]. In practice, so that we do not have to deal with squares, we more often use the square root of variance which is called the **standard deviation**[2] (σ or **SD**). This has the same units as the mean as opposed to units squared, as is the case with variance. The standard deviation relates to the variation (dispersion) of the data. If the data are equally distributed, one may obtain a better understanding of data points by using SD. In the usual normal distribution, the data that lie within one SD from the mean encompass about 2/3 of all data points; the data that lie within two SD from the mean represent 95% of all data points and the data that lie within three SD from the mean contain 99% of all data points.

---

[1]The reason is complex and beyond the scope of this text. However, in an oversimplified way, it has to do with the fact that for a given sum if you know n – 1 you could predict the nth factor, so that n – 1 represents the independent findings that determine the variance

[2]The symbols for mean and standard deviation vary in most texts. Classically, $\bar{x}$ or μ are used for the mean of the entire population, and x for that of a group. Similarly σ is used for the standard deviation of the entire population, and s for the standard deviation of a group

Furthermore, if we know for a given data point how many SD it is away from the mean $[Xi - \bar{x}]/SD = z$, then we could identify what percentage of observations lie above or below this data point (see Appendix I for z values).

As an example, if for a certain group the mean serum cholesterol (x) is 200 and the SD is 30 then an individual [Xi] with a cholesterol value of 250 has a z distribution of ($[250 - 200]/30 = 1.66$) and is 1.66 standard deviations away from the mean. Looking at Appendix I, we see this implies that 4.85% of this group has a higher cholesterol and 95.15% has a lower cholesterol than 250. This is shown schematically in Figure 2.

It is apparent, therefore, that if we know the mean and the standard deviation of a value within a population, we could then predict the probability that a given value is part of such a population. It is also understood that this is applicable only in populations with normal (Gaussian)[3] distribution, where the mean is approximately the point with most observations and the data around the mean are distributed equally.

Another often used measure of variation is the **coefficient of variation** (CV) in which the standard deviation is expressed as a percentage of the mean. As opposed to the standard deviation,which is an absolute measure of variability around the mean, the coefficient of variation (a dimensionless unit) allows for determination of relative variability around the mean. It has the advantage that it permits comparison of groups with analogous characteristics. For instance, if the blood pressure of a geriatric population is 110 ± 10 mmHg (mean $\pm$ SD) then CV is about 9%. One may compare that with normal pregnant women with a mean pressure of 70 ± 6 and a CV again of 9% (a similar data variation). Another important feature of CV is that it allows some conclusions regarding the data distribution. A CV less than 10% suggests tight data, while values in excess of 40% suggest substantial scatter and possibly a skewed distribution.

Two more coefficients exist that describe the shape of distribution of data. The first is the **coefficient of skewness**[4]. In simple terms, in the normal (Gaussian) distribution, the mean is the same as the median and the mode and is represented by a smooth symmetrical curve without a one-sided tail. If there is a tail to the left (if the mean is to the left of the median and the mode) the distribution is said to be negatively skewed. In the opposite case (tail to the right and mean to the right of median and mode) we have a positive skew. The other coefficient that deals with the shape of the distribution curve is the **coefficient of kurtosis**[5]. This deals

---

[3]From the name of the German mathematician, Frederick Gauss, normal distribution is also called Bell-shape curve to allow for a pictorial visualization of the distribution
[4]Coefficient of skewness $= \sum (y - y)^3/s^3$. s = standard deviation
[5]Coefficient of kurtosis $= \sum (y - y)^4/s^4$

Total population

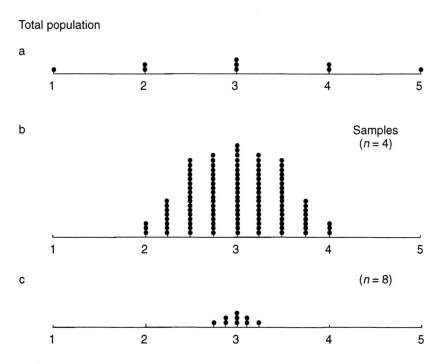

Figure 3 Examples of distribution and sample size and their effects on mean values and standard deviations

with the relative height of the peak of the distribution. A normal distribution has a coefficient of 3. Less than 3 indicates a thin-pointed curve (leptokurtosis), while a value higher than 3 suggests a broad curve (platykurtosis).

Let us now deal with samples from a given population rather than the entire population. For purposes of demonstration we will consider an unusually small population of only 9 data points: 1, 2, 2, 3, 3, 3, 4, 4, 5 (Figure 3a). The mean is 3, and the standard deviation is 1.15 suggesting that almost all (95% or 2 standard deviations) values of such a population will be between 0.70 and 5.3. Now, consider different sample sizes and their mean. If we first consider samples of $n = 4$, then the smallest possible combination (1, 2, 2, 3) will have a mean of 2 and a highest possible combination (3, 4, 4 and 5) will have a mean of 4. If the means of all possible combinations are plotted, a new distribution will be produced, again with a mean of 3 but with a smaller range, 2 to 4 (Figure 3b), and as a result a smaller standard deviation of 0.57. Finally if we have a larger sample size, say $n = 8$, an even tighter population distribution range will be encountered (2.75 to 3.25) while the mean will remain at 3 (Figure

3c). It is apparent that using samples of larger sizes does not allow random means to deviate far from the actual mean of the total population. The standard deviation of means of samples is called the **standard error of mean** (SEM) and can be calculated by dividing the standard deviation of a sample by the square root of the number of observation of the sample, $SD/\sqrt{n}$.

Note that the standard deviation allows conclusions to be drawn concerning data points relative to the population. In essence it answers the question: what is the likelihood that a data point with a value x is part of the population? In the initial example, if the height of 12-year-old girls is 155 ± 5 cm (mean $\pm$ SD), one appreciates that 140 cm is 3 SD away from the mean. Thus a girl with a height 140 cm has a chance of about 0.5% (or 1 in 200) to be encountered in this population. If indeed she is part of the population she will then qualify as an extreme member (short stature). The standard error of mean (SEM) answers a totally different question; what is the likelihood that the mean of a class of 25 girls in the 6th grade (12 years old) will have a height of 150 cm?

Since SEM $= SD/\sqrt{n} = 5/\sqrt{25} = 1$ then the height of the 12-year-old girls could be described as 150 ± 1 cm (mean $\pm$ SEM). As previously stated, SEM is the standard deviation of the distribution of all possible means of 25 subjects. We may then say, for example, that 150 is 5 SEMs away from the population mean (since SEM $= 1$ cm) and thus such a group is not likely to derive from the usual population. The number of SEMs by which one sample mean differs from the population mean is called t and is analogous to z ($t =$ distance from $\bar{x}/$SEM). The reason that t is higher than z, even though in essence t and z deal with the similar determination, is the fact that we usually deal with a small sample size (or number of subjects). Note in Appendix II that as the sample size approaches infinity then $t = z$.

It is common for a statistican to describe data with confidence intervals (CI). By that they mean the range in which one would expect the mean of a sample to be included. As you may have predicted, for continuous data:

$$95\% \text{ CI} = \text{mean} \pm (t_{0.05}) \text{ SEM}$$
$$\text{and} \quad 99\% \text{ CI} = \text{mean} \pm (t_{0.01}) \text{ SEM}$$

For the height data these translate into

$$95\% \text{ CI} = 150 \pm 2.06 \times 1$$
$$99\% \text{ CI} = 150 \pm 2.79 \times 1$$

In other words, a sample of 25 girls of that age group should have a mean between 147.94 and 152.06 in 95% of such samples. You may recognize that t and CI represent the basis for comparison of population means (inferential analysis – see next Chapter).

ORDINAL DATA

As we said before, use of continuous data and analysis of their central tendency and dispersions by using mean and standard error of mean is applicable only when data are distributed normally[6]. The predictions we described before, for instance confidence intervals, cannot be used for skewed populations. Indeed, use of mean and standard deviations or standard error of mean are inappropriate to describe such distributions. Transformation of data to the natural logarithmic (ln x) or inverse form ($1/x$) may switch the data to a normal distribution and thus allow use of statistical analysis as already described. However, it is probably better if in doubt to use the **median** (the level of the $n/2$th value) for the central tendency and use quartiles (25%, 75%) or range to describe dispersion. For instance, if a group is composed of 1, 2, 3, 10 , one could rank them from the smallest (1) to the largest (10, 4th value). The median is then 2.5 (between 2 and 3) and the range is between 1 and 10.

NOMINAL DATA

As stated in the introduction, data may also be nominal. For example, a tuberculin test is either positive or negative, or a person may be dead or alive, thin or obese. Here the presentation of data is either in the form of rates (1 per 1000 men) or percentages (i.e. 10%). Obviously, higher rates are shown as percentages. Let us consider a group of people, say workers of a certain company who have had a tuberculin test. Let us also say that 281 out of 1411 workers had a positive tuberculin test. One may then say that about 20% of workers (281/1411) had come in contact with tuberculosis. If we take samples of this population, say groups of 5, it appears likely that the average group will have 1 person positive out of 5 (20%) although there will be groups with either 0 out of 5 (0%) or 2, 3 or more (40%, 60% or more respectively) (Figure 4a). If we move to groups of 20, the average group will contain 4 positive workers although higher or lower rates will be also encountered (Figure 4b). You recognize however that having 0 or 12 subjects positive (0% and 60% respectively) is rather unlikely with such a sizable group. If we further increase the size of the group, then the positive responses will be clustered around the expected one. Indeed, notice that the distribution approaches what we have already described for normal distribution in the continuous data. Therefore,

---

[6]Normal distribution typically predicts that the proportion of a given value is predicted from its z, that is to say the number of standard deviations away from the mean by
$$y = 0.3989 \ e^{-z^2/2}$$
In a more simplified expression a distribution is called normal if its mean is about equal to its median (no outliers) and mode (no bimodal distribution)

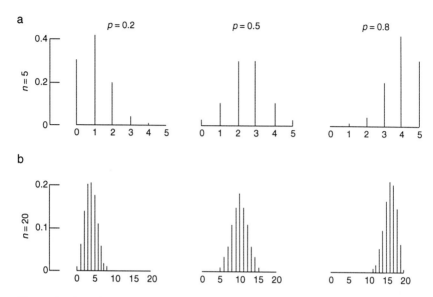

Figure 4   Distribution of nominal data (see text)

under those conditions, the data may be described as mean percent ± SEM (SEM = $\sqrt{p(1-p)}/n$, where p equals the probabilty, i.e.0.6 for 60%. We all know that during elections statisticians poll a sample of the population and indicate that candidate X is supported by 40% (i.e. 40% of subjects questioned). They also give you a range – usually ± 2SEM. For example, if 40 out of 100 support candidate A, the mean will be 40% with a standard error of mean of about 5 ($\sqrt{40 \times 60}/100$), so the expected actual support is between 30 and 50% ($40 \pm 2 \times 5$). If the same result came out of a sample of 1000 people then S = $\sqrt{40 \times 60}/1000$ or about 1.5 and his actual support will be between 37 and 43%, a much tighter prediction.

Occasionally, nominal events happen at very low rates, making it difficult to present proportions in a meaningful way. For instance, 325 patients with nephrolithiasis required a total of 615 hospitalizations in 5 years. The best way to express this nominal event is as a rate, i.e. the chance for hospitalization for a nephrolithiasis patient is, on average 615/325 = 1.89 times in a 5-year span. Although the probability is that such a patient will be hospitalized twice in this time interval, the possibility exists that he/she may be hospitalized once, three or five times. The distribution of such probabilities is called the **Poisson distribution** and has the following formulation:

$$P(x) = \frac{\lambda^x e^{-\lambda}}{x!}$$

Where $P(x)$ is the probability the event will occur x times, λ (the Greek letter lambda) is the average rate (mean), e is the base of the natural

Table 2   Probabilities for Poisson Distribution with $\lambda = 1.89$

Number of Hospitalizations (x)	1.89^x	$e^{-1.89}$	$x!$	$P(x)$
0	1	0.15	1	0.15
1	1.89	0.15	1	0.29
2	3.57	0.15	2	0.27
3	6.78	0.15	6	0.17
4	12.76	0.15	24	0.08
5	24.12	0.15	120	0.03
6	45.58	0.15	720	0.01

Table 3   Comparison of the characteristics of binomial and Poisson distributions

	Binomial	*Poisson*
Probability of event	p	p
Probability of no event	$1-p$	1
Variance	$p(1-p)$	p
Standard Deviation	$\sqrt{p(1-p)}$	$\sqrt{p}$
Standard Error of Mean	$\sqrt{p(1-p)/n}$	$\sqrt{p/n}$

logarithm, and $x!$ is the factorial value of x. The Poisson distribution[7] is used to predict the probability that a given event will occur. For instance, what is the probability that a patient with nephrolithiasis will need four admissions?

$$P(4) = \frac{1.89^4 e^{-1.89}}{4!} = \frac{12.76 \times 0.15}{24} = 0.08$$

i.e. it has an 8% chance. Table 2 shows the probabilities for hospitalization for Poisson distribution with $\lambda = 1.89$. Figure 5 schematically depicts this distribution.

As in binomial distribution, Poisson distribution also has a distribution that approaches normal. However, if the probability of an event is very small, the probability of an event *not* happening is infinitely higher. As shown in Table 3, this results in a variance equal to the mean and a standard deviation equal to the square root of the mean probability. Thus the 95% confidence interval for such a probability will equal $p \pm 1.96 \sqrt{p}$.

---

[7]After the French mathematician, Simeon-Denis Poisson who deduced it in 1837

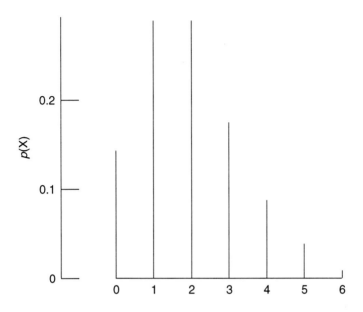

Figure 5 Graphical representation of the data in Table 2

RATES

If a portion of the population develops a given characteristic over a time interval (occurrences/population), this proportion is called the **rate**. This proportion needs not to be expressed as a percentage, but as cases per population size. If we deal with new phenomena (occurrences) over a period of time, this rate is called **incidence**. For example, let us consider the situation where we encounter 862 cases of myocardial infarction (MI) in a group of 10 000 retired officers in 2 years. One may express the incidence as 431 MI per 10 000 officers per year. Notice, there is nothing special about the denominator (10 000). The incidence will be expressed equally well if we say 43.1MI per 1000 officers per year or that 4.31% of officers developed MI in a year period. On the other hand, if we care about the proportion of the population that has a given disease at a specified point in time, this rate is called **prevalence**.

A combination of proportions and rates is often helpful to allow one to find how likely a characteristic is expected to occur in a given group. **Relative risk** is ratio of the incidence of an occurrence in one group relative to the incidence in another (often control) group. For instance, if the incidence of a given disease is 20% in smokers, as opposed to only 4% in non-smokers, one will calculate relative risk of 20/4 = 5. That is to say the relative risk is 5 times higher for people who smoke. A similar index is the **odds ratio**. In the odds ratio, we compare the ratio of diseased versus

19

non-diseased in one group against a similar ratio in the other group. In the example we just dealt with the odds ratio will be $(20/80)/(4/96) = 6$, not terribly different from the ratio we found for the relative risk.

PROBABILITIES

Probability is the chance an event has to occur in a given population. The reason we described data distribution above was to find the probability of a given data sum or event to occur. In our first example (Figure 2), the probability that one has high cholesterol (identified arbitrarily as a level above 250) is 5%. In our other example, the probability that a given individual has a positive tuberculin test is 20%. An important calculation is that of the probability of a given individual having both a high cholesterol and a positive tuberculin test. This is equal to p (high cholesterol) × p (positive tuberculin) = 5% × 20% = 1%. The reason we multiply is simple. Think of 100 workers, then 20 will have positive tuberculin. From those 20 only 5% (1 in 20) is expected to have high cholesterol. Therefore only 1 out of 100 is expect to have both. The importance of such calculations is significant epidemiologically. Another probability one may elect to calculate is that of having either a morbid condition (either high cholesterol or a positive tuberculin test). In this case the probability of a morbid event will equal the probability of one event (high cholesterol) plus the probability of the other event (positive tuberculin test) minus the probability of both. The reason for subtracting the combination group is that they have already been accounted for as members of each group. In our example this will be $0.20 + 0.05 - 0.01 = 0.24$, or 24%. You would have come to the same conclusion if you did the calculations simplistically. In such a case, 20 workers have high cholesterol, and of the remaining 80, about 5%, i.e. 4, will have positive PPD $(20 + 4 = 24\%)$.

The examples we just mentioned dealt with probabilities that are independent of each other. However, sometimes we deal with probabilities that are mutually exclusive. For instance one may have only one blood types (A, B, O, or AB). In such a case, the question could be asked: what is the probability of blood type A or B in a population? This is essentially the same as above $p(\text{A or B}) = p(\text{A}) + p(\text{B})$, but of course without the factor $p(\text{A and B})$ since, unlike cholesterol and +PPD, it is not possible to be both blood type A and blood type B. Table 4 shows all the equations used for probabilities.

A more complex situation (but clinically far more important) is the so called Bayesian analysis[8]. In this approach the probability of a given disease

---

[8]Thomas Bayes, an Englishman, described it but was hesitant to publish because of the complexities of the assumptions made. The essay was published by a friend in 1763 after his death

Table 4   Probability formulae

Sample Probability

$$p \, (\text{event}) = \frac{\text{number of events}}{\text{number of observations}}$$

Combination Probabilities

1. Independent events

   (a) All events to happen
       p (event 1 + event 2 + ...) = p (event 1) × p (event 2) ....

   (b) Any event to happen
       p (event 1 or event 2) = p (event 1) + p (event 2) – P (event 1 + event 2)

2. Conditional probabilities

   (a) p (event E, given a certain condition C) = p (E/C)
   (b) Combinations of events/conditions (Bayes' formula)

   $$p(E_1 / C) = \frac{p(E_1) \times p(C / E_1)}{p(E_1) \times p(C / E_1) + p(E_2) \times p(C / E_2)...}$$

---

before analysis is called the **prior probability**. This is modified according to conditional probabilities, that is to say the chance that a given symptom or finding is likely to occur with such a disease. The final, **posterior probability**, what actually leads to our diagnosis. Let us consider chest pain in a 60-year-old man without evidence of trauma or pneumonia. Let us also assume that myocardial infarction and angina pectoris (MI) account for 80% of such cases, pulmonary embolism (PE) accounts for 5% and pericarditis (PC) for the remaining 5%. Let us then deal with three different clinical presentations. Patient A is in end-stage renal disease, with pain that is modified with position, is preload dependent (blood pressure drops with minimal fluid renewal during dialysis) and ST segment elevation in the electrcardiogram (EKG). Patient B had a car accident, hip surgery and is immobilized in a cast, and has chest pain that is in pleuritic in nature. Patient C has diaphoresis, ST elevation and diffuse atherosclerosis.

Table 5 used the Bayes' formula and identified a different posterior probability for each patient, depending on his clinical picture (and conditional probabilities). You may appreciate that the findings are consistent with clinical diagnosis of pericarditis in patient A, pulmonary embolism in patient B, and myocardial infarction in patient C. In essence we all do a similar analysis in our brains, even though more simplistically. The way that one actually performs this analysis is to take the prior probability for each disease $p(D1)$, $p(D2)$ . . . and the conditional

Table 5 Use of Bayes' formula in calculating probabilities. Details of abbreviations are given in the text

Prior probabilities	Conditional probabilities – p(C/E)				Posterior probabilities
	Renal failure	Positional	Pre-load dependence	ST elevation	
MI 0.80	0.30	0.02	0.10	0.80	0.0216
PE 0.15	0.10	0.05	0.10	0.01	< 0.001
PC 0.05	0.60	0.80	0.90	0.90	0.925
	Hip surgery	Immobilization	Pleuritic		
MI 0.80	0.10	0.01	0.01		0.0012
PE 0.15	0.50	0.80	0.80		0.9983
PC 0.05	0.01	0.01	0.10		< 0.001
	ST elevation	Diaphoresis	ASCVD		
MI 0.80	0.80	0.80	0.90		0.9999
PE 0.15	0.01	0.10	0.01		< 0.001
PC 0.05	0.80	0.10	0.01		< 0.001

Bayes' formula

$$p(D_1/F) = \frac{p(D_1) \times p(F/D_1)}{p(D_1) \times p(F/D_1) + p(D_2) \times p(F/D_2)...}$$

Where $p(D_1)$ is the probability of disease 1 (prior)
$p(F/D_1)$ is the probability of a finding in patients with 1 disease (conditional probability)
note: The conditional probabilities are for the most part hypothetical, not exact findings of any study

probability of the symptom or sign $p(F/D1)$, $p(F/D2)$ . . . , put them in the formula shown in Table 5 and identify a new probability. This new probability is then used instead of the prior probability as we move to the second conditional probability and so forth, till we exhaust all conditional probabilities. The final such probability is called the **posterior probability** and represents the chance of this disease based on the likelihood of the finding for each disease (**conditional probability**). For instance, given chest pain and the clinical findings in patient A, the chance he has pericarditis is 0.975 (97.5%) while that of MI is only 2.16%. By contrast in patient B, the chance he has pulmonary embolism is 99.8% and in patient C, it is almost certain he has an MI (99.9%)

ODDS RATIO

The probability of a given event or finding to happen, can also be expressed as a ratio of the odds that this event will likely happen relative to the odds that it will not happen. In other words the probability that chest pain in a 60-year-old is 80% to be indicative of coronary ischemia, it may be presented as a chance of 4:1 to be due to ischemia, since he has a probability of 80% to be ischemic in origin, and 20% to be non-ischemic (80/20 = 4). This ratio is called the **odds ratio**, and we will deal with it in some depth in the next chapter. The **odds ratio (OR)** can be determined from the probability p and vice versa, as OR = $p/(1-p)$, or p = OR/(1 + OR). The advantage of the odds ratio is that it may simplify the rather complex calculations we encountered before, as we were dealing with probabilities. We may rewrite the Bayes' theorem using LR and OR to read: post-test odds = pre-test odds × likelihood ratio. **Likelihood ratio** (LR) is the ratio of the probability of a finding in the condition of interest relative to the probability of the same finding in all the other conditions encountered. For instance, the presence of diaphoresis makes the likelihood ratio 4, i.e. the ratio of the probability that diaphoresis occurs in a patient with MI over the possibility that diaphoresis occurs in the two other conditions considered in Table 5 (0.8/0.2). Thus the initial OR of 4 (for a probability of 0.8) will produce a new OR of 16 that corresponds with a probability of 0.94 (16/17). Stated differently, a 60-year-old with chest pain and diaphoresis has a 16:1 chance to have an ischemic event, or 94% probability.

The transformation of probabilities to ratios becomes reasonably easy with practice. The recently fashionable **evidence-based medicine** emphasizes the use of the modified Bayes' theorem in an effort to identify more objectively the likelihood of a given disease given the existing data, or to identify the likelihood of a given therapeutic regimen. Further manipulations of the odds ratio for a given test or therapeutic regimen will allow one to find how many patients will be needed to have a positive test or to be treated with a given drug to ensure a definite success over not performing such a test or treatment with this therapy. This part of evidence-based medicine is discussed in more detail in Chapter 7.

Before closing this chapter, it is necessary to identify possible shortcommings from the use of the evidence-based medicine. By far the more important source of error is the use of erroneous probabilities and ratios. One has to be extremely careful in obtaining such informations from the existing literature. For instance, if a paper suggests that two out of four patients with pneumonia expired when treated with the usual antibiotics, one shall not consider a $p = 0.5$ in making deductions regarding the prognosis of a given patient or the therapeutic superiority of a new antibiotic. This is because the number of patients is **particularly** small and does not exclude with confidence that the actual death rate of the entire population may actually be as low as 10% or as high as 90%, as we discussed earlier in this Chapter. The quality of the study is of outmost importance. If a study is prospective it is certainly far more believable than a retrospective one. The presence of bias shall be looked for very carefully. For example the findings on pneumonia in residents of a nursing home for the elderly, will have little relevance, if any, regarding young individuals with AIDS and pneumonia. All these issues, and more, are discussed in some detail in the final chapter. Another important point deserves re-emphasis. This has to do with the presentation of the data. It is commonplace for a test to be categorized as positive or negative. It was emphasized earlier (Chapter 1) that data shall not be presented as categorical if they could be presented as continuous, or even ordinal. For example, the chances that the middle age man with substernal chest pain has MI are more if his CK-MB is very high, rather than when it is hardly detectable. Similarly, a patient with a non-positive lung scan may have less chances of having her pulmonary embolism identified compared to being classified in an ordinal fashon, and have her test interpreted as of intermediate probability (instead of non-positive).

TAKE HOME MESSAGES

- Identify the average of a given group as either the **mean** (continuous and nominal data) or **median** (ordinal data).
- Identify a measure of dispersion of data around the mean as **standard deviation**, SD (continuous and nominal data), **range**, or **quartiles** (ordinal data).
- Standard error of mean, SEM, represents the standard deviation of means of a given sample size (n).
- The probability that a given data point is part of a population is determined by the number of SD that the data point is away from the population mean (z).

- The probability that a given sample is part a population is determined by the number of SEM the sample's mean is away from the population's mean (t).
- The probability that two or more situations could take place simultaneously can be computed. It is the combinations of the probabilities of symptoms, signs and laboratory findings that will lead to identification of a condition (i.e. disease) that is likely to occur, or not.
- Possibilities can be transformed to odds ratio as OR = $p/(1-p)$.
- Likelihood ratio is the ratio that compares the probability of a given finding in the condition under consideration versus the probability of this finding in all other conditions.
- Post test OR = pre-test OR × likelihood ratio.

QUESTIONS

1. If the mean hematocrit in a normal healthy adult women is 42 and the standard deviation is 2.5:
   (a) What is the normal range (i.e. one that includes 95% of normal adult women)?
   (b) A woman was found to have a hematocrit of 39. Is that considered normal?
   (c) The average hematocrit of a group of women ($n = 25$) is 39. Is this considered normal?
2. In a final examination in physiology given to 100 medical students, the average student scored 64 (out of 100). The standard deviation was 8.
   (a) Where shall we set the pass mark to have 80% of the medical students pass the test?
   (b) If the passing mark was set at 60, how many students will pass this exam?
3. Five percent of pregnant women are found to have urinary tract infection during the first prenatal visit. Of those labeled as normal, about 5% will develop urinary tract infection during their pregnancy. What is the overall percentage of women having urinary tract infection at some time during pregnancy?
4. A patient develops acute renal failure and oliguria. His urine analysis shows granular casts and a urine Na$^+$ of 50 mEq/l. Presume we are considering only the diagnoses of pre-renal acute renal failure (PR) and acute tubular necrosis (ATN). Granular casts are seen in 75% of patients with ATN, and only 1% in those with PR. Also, urine Na$^+$ higher than 20 mEq/l is seen in 95% of patients with ATN, and 2% of those with PR. It is felt that ATN and PR have an equal chance to develop, given the underlying condition of the patient. Based on

this patient's urinary findings, what is the probability that this patient has ATN?

5. In an average day, 5 patients of a hemodialysis unit are in-patient. The chief of nephrology likes to have most of these cases admitted into the nephrology ward.

   (a) How many beds should he/she request from the administrator of the hospital for this reason?

   (b) How likely is it to have 10 hemodialysis patients as in-patients in a given day?

   (c) What about 2 hemodialysis patients?

6. The complication rate of a surgical procedure is 20%. When you review the charts of 20 patients who had such an operation, you find that 10 patients had complications. Is there a suggestion of possible problems with this procedure in your institution?

CHAPTER 3

Inferential statistics – the basics

SENSITIVITY, SPECIFICITY, PREDICTIVE VALUES

Formulation of data, as we have shown in the previous Chapter, allows some deduction based on the probability of a particular data point occurring. For instance, for the group of men with cholesterol levels of 200 ± 30 mg/dl (mean $\pm$ SD), we determined that levels over 250 mg/dl occur in less than 5% of the population. It appears logical, therefore, to use 250 as the cut off above which a person is labeled as hypercholesterolemic. If we use atherosclerotic disease as a measure of pathology due to high cholesterol, we may find that 90% of atherosclerotic patients had levels over 250 mg/dl, while only 5% of those without atherosclerosis had that high a value. Note, that if we lower the cut off for hypercholesterolemia, more of the atherosclerotic patients (true positives) will be included (higher sensitivity) but this will result in a higher percentage of normals (false positives) being included (lower specificity), see Figure 6.

As you may have recognized from the above, the **sensitivity** of a test is the percentage of actually diseased people identified as positive by this test. **Specificity**, on the other hand, is a measure of the ability of the test to discriminate between diseased and normal. The percentage of normal subjects with a negative test represents such a discriminatory function (Table 6).

In addition, **the predictive value of a positive test** (i.e. the probability of obtaining a positive test in diseased individuals), and **the predictive value of a negative test** (i.e. the probability of getting a negative test in normal subjects) are also significant components used to describe the significance of a test. The relative importance of specificity, sensitivity and the predictive value of a positive or negative test is determined by two factors: (1) the prevalence of the disease, and (2) the reasons the test is used (i.e. screening to identify the diseased versus screening to exclude the normal individuals). Let us briefly address these issues.

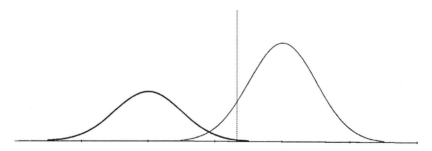

Figure 6 Distribution of cholesterol levels in subjects with and without atherosclerosis. For details see text

Table 6 Diagramatic representation of the concepts sensitivity, specificity, and predictive value

Test	DISEASE Present	Absent	
Positive	a	b	a + b, All subjects with positive test
Negative	c	d	c + d, All subjects with negative test
	a + c	b + d	
	all diseased	all normal	

SENSITIVITY Proportion of subject with disease that have positive test (positive in disease)

$$\frac{a}{a + c}$$

SPECIFICITY Proportion of normal that have a negative test (negative in health)

$$\frac{d}{b + d}$$

PREDICTIVE VALUE OF A POSITIVE TEST Proportion of diseased subjects among those that develop a positive test

$$\frac{a}{a + b}$$

PREDICTIVE VALUE OF A NEGATIVE TEST Proportion of normal subject among those that have a negative test

$$\frac{d}{c + d}$$

Table 7 Predictive value of a positive test in a population with a low prevalence (a) or a high prevalence (b)

Test	Diseased		Normal
(a)			
Positive	99	99	198
Negative	1	9801	9802
Total	100	9900	10 000
(b)			
Positive	4950	50	5000
Negative	50	4950	5000
Total	5000	5000	10 000

First, consider two groups of prospective blood donors – one composed of mostly middle-class people from the mid-West, and the other a group of people from the inner city with a high percentage of intravenous drug abusers. The expected incidence of AIDS is about 1% in the first group and 50% in the second group. Let us consider that a test (say ELISA for HIV) has a sensitivity of 99% and a specificity of 99%. As shown in Table 7, a positive test represents many false-positive subjects in the first group while it represents mostly diseased people in the second group. Thus prevalence is related closely to the predictive value of a positive test for any level of sensitivity and specificity of a given test (Figure 7).

As we mentioned before, changing the cut off to increase the sensitivity will reduce specificity and therefore increase the rate of false positive tests. The curve that describes such a relationship is called the receiver-operated control curve (ROC curve, Figure 8). Note that the straight line indicates a ROC of a test with no discriminatory value, thus called the indifference line. A good ROC is when the surface between the curve and the line of indifference is large. In other words, the larger the surface area of the ROC, the better, that is, the more discriminatory a test is. You may remember from Chapter 2 that the likelihood ratio of a test is the ratio of the probability of a positive result in subjects that have a given disease (sensitivity) over the probability for a positive test to be present in subjects that do not have this disease (false positive). In short, ROC is a graphic representation of the likelihood ratio. It is apparent that a high likelihood ratio, that is the best cut off point for a test, is the point closer to the corner. This represents the best sensitivity to false positive ratio that allows one to have the highest possible sensitivity. ROC curves have a dual advantage. For one they allow an immediate optical evaluation of the validity of a test. In addition, they permit identification of the appropriate cut off for a given test. That is why they became so common in the recent literature.

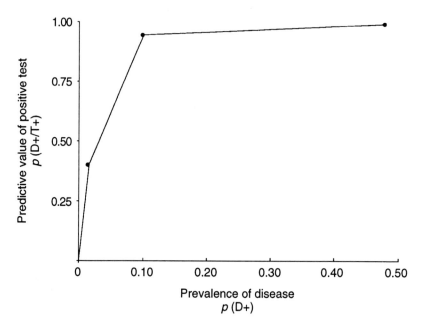

Figure 7   Role of prevalence of a given disease to influence the predictive value of a positive test. In a disease with low prevalence, a positive test is of limited significance

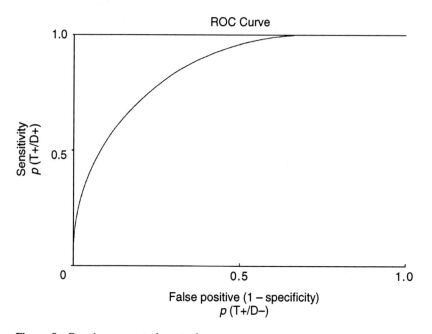

Figure 8   Receiver-operated control curve

STATISTICAL ERRORS

A similar situation is encountered when two groups of subjects are evaluated with regard to a test that is expressed in continuous data. Let us compare, for instance the level of uric acid in two groups of pregnant women, normal and pre-eclamptic (Figure 9). The mean of the normal pregnant women is substantially lower than that of pre-eclamptic patients. As in most biological phenomena, this is not a black and white situation and overlap occurs.

So, for any cut off point, those in a certain percentage of normals will have uric acid level higher than that point (α value) and a portion of pre-eclamptics will have a lower level (β value). Similarly to the case of sensitivity, the more one moves the cut off in order to decrease α, the less it is likely that a point beyond α belongs to the group under consideration. However, β increases making it more likely for data from the opposite group to be considered part of the first group. In practice, we use the complementary of β, the **power**. Conventionally, an α of 0.05 and a β of 0.2 (power = $1 - \beta = 0.8$) is selected as a cut off to allow for a meaningful discrimination between the two groups.

When comparing two groups, we first assume that there is no real difference between them, and that they represent random samples of the overall population. We then evaluate the chance that this basic hypothesis (**null hypothesis**) is true. If this has a very low probability, ($p < 0.05$) we then reject the null hypothesis and conclude that the two groups originate from separate populations, and that they are statistically significantly different. The chance the two groups are, in fact, part of a single population is 5% or less; i.e. only a 1 in 20 chance exists (5%) that the two samples originate from the same population. Note, however, that there

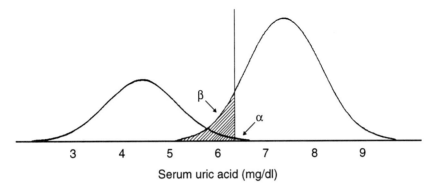

Serum uric acid (mg/dl)

Figure 9 Serum uric acid in normal and pre-eclamptic pregnant women. The vertical line at 6.5 mg/dl represents the cut off to separate normal from high levels. Note that above 6.5 mg/dl there are few normal pregnant women α error). Similarly they are few pre-eclamptic patients with a normal uric acid level (β error)

31

Table 8 Factors influencing decision making in testing a hypothesis

	Actual situation	
	Real difference	*No difference*
Difference present	Power $(1 - \beta)$	Type I error (α error)
No difference	Type II error (β error)	$1 - \alpha$

is still a possibility (5%) that we have made an error in rejecting the hypothesis, a so-called alpha (α) or Type I error. This is called α error because we could have prevented it if we had selected a more conservative α, say 0.01 that allows $p < 0.01$ to discriminate between acceptance and rejection of the null hypothesis.

It is particularly important to use a low α level if the expected difference between groups is small. For example, let us first consider two groups, one with cholesterol of 250 ± 30 mg/dl (a group of nephrotic patients) and a second, control group with a cholesterol of 180 ± 30 mg/dl and say that they have a $p < 0.05$. In such a case the two groups appear quite different, and thus the finding of a statistically significant difference appears consistent with our impression. Now let us consider two other groups, one with a cholesterol of 185 ± 2 mg/dl versus a control group with 180 ± 2 mg/dl again, with a $p < 0.05$. In this case, the small difference between the groups raises the possibility that we are actually getting extreme cases of the same population, therefore erroneously depicting the populations as different, when in reality they are not. Obviously, no discriminating evaluator (reader, editor, etc.) will be impressed or accept such a difference as real. If one wishes to assert such a conclusion then a much tighter difference, such as $p < 0.001$ may be necessary. Even then, one may say that it passed the p test, but failed the 'so what' test!

On the other hand, if we have two groups with cholesterol 350 ± 60 versus 180 ± 50 mg/dl that do not reach statistical significance, the problem may lie in the fact that there are a limited number of observations. This results in the extreme values giving a substantial variance within the groups that does not permit the conclusion that the groups are different, when in fact they may be. If a larger sample is selected, the variance may decrease and the beta (β) overlap percentage will decrease (or $1-\beta$, the power, will increase). The type of error whereby a real difference is not revealed is called a beta (β) or Type II error, see Table 8.

NUMBER OF SUBJECTS NEEDED IN A STUDY

Implicit in the previous analysis is that appropriate selection of α and β is necessary to allow one to draw the 'correct' conclusion relative to statistical

Table 9 Number of subjects (K) needed to obtain significant differences (see text)

Significance (α)	Power (1 − β)	K
0.05	0.99	18.372
	0.95	12.995
	0.90	10.502
	0.80	7.849
0.01	0.99	24.031
	0.95	17.814
	0.90	14.879
	0.80	11.679

differences. The other major determinant of statistical differences in addition to α and β is the number of subjects (n). A close relationship among all these factors exists, and they can be used prospectively to predict the n needed for a study, given the accepted levels of α, β, the expected difference, Δ, and the variability of the population (standard deviation, SD, σ).

In the case of two groups:

$$n = 2\left[\frac{(Z\alpha - Z\beta)\sigma}{\Delta}\right]^2$$

where $Z\alpha$ is the z for $\alpha = 0.05$ (1.96 see Appendix I) and $Z\beta$ for $\beta = 0.20$, (or power of 0.8) is −0.85. To simplify matters the equation could be transformed to

$$n = \frac{K \times 2\sigma^2}{\Delta^2}$$

where K could be found from Table 9 for any level of significance (α) and power $(1 - \beta)$ usually considered for studies.

For example, if we plan to evaluate the effectiveness of a new antihypertensive and will accept a difference of 10 mmHg of the hypertensive's blood pressure as a minimum of effectiveness ($\Delta = 10$), assume a standard deviation of 5 mmHg ($\sigma = 10$) and elect $\alpha = 0.05$, and $1 - \beta = 0.8$ then the number of participants in each group should be

$$n = \frac{7.85 \times 2 \times 10^2}{10^2} = 15.70 \text{ or } 16 \text{ subjects}$$

A similar situation exist for proportions. Let us assume that patients in the intensive care unit with pseudomonas bacteremia have a survival rate of 50% with the present antibiotic regimen. We are about to consider a new antibiotic and say we will accept an increase in survival of at least 10% as our cut off before we approve this antibiotic. You probably remember that in the case of a proportion, the standard deviation equals $\sqrt{p(1-p)}$. Since we have two proportions then the average standard deviation will equal the average of the two standard deviations, i.e.

$$\sqrt{\left[p_1(1-p_1)+p_2(1-p_2)\right]/2}$$

In our example

$$n = \frac{7.85 \times 2 \times \left[\sqrt{(0.05 \times 0.5)+(0.6 \times 0.4)/2}\right]^2}{0.1^2}$$

$$= \frac{7.85 \times 2 \times \left[(0.5 \times 0.5)+(0.6 \times 0.4)/2\right]}{0.1^2} = 384 \text{ subjects to each group}$$

Finally, the number of subjects needed to identify a true linear regression could also be identified by a similar equation.

BASIC CONCEPTS INVOLVED IN COMPARISON OF GROUPS

In inferential statistics we examine whether two or more groups are derived from the same population. For that, we identify the difference between the groups (Δ mean) and the confidence limits of the difference, similar to the procedure described for the distribution of a single group. For a large number of observations ($n > 60$) this could be described as:

confidence limits = Δ mean $\pm$ Z SEM

and for

95% confidence limits = Δ mean $\pm$ 1.96 SEM

For smaller size groups this is modified to

confidence limits = Δ mean $\pm$ t_n SEM

where t is found for $n - 1$ degrees of freedom from Appendix II.

If zero (0) is included within the confidence limits we conclude that no difference is very likely and thus accept the null hypothesis. In contrast, if zero is outside the confidence limits, we then assert the possibility that the two groups are similar, and thus it is highly unlikely that they are derived from a single population. In such a case we assume that the two groups are statistically different from each other. Alternatively we can solve for z (if $n > 60$) or t (if $n < 60$) as follows:

$$z, t = \frac{\Delta \text{ mean}}{\text{SEM}}$$

and check z or t in Appendices I or II, respectively, to find the level of probability that the two groups are part of a single population. In either case the higher the difference and/or the less the variance, the more one is convinced that the two groups are different from each other.

If more than two groups are involved, it appears more complex to identify whether a given group belongs to a different population. It is easily understood that if 20 groups are compared there is a one in twenty chance that one will differ (< 0.05), even if they derive from the same population. In such cases we first evaluate the variability of the means of the group versus the variability of the overall data by a technique known as analysis of variance (ANOVA) where

$$F = \frac{\text{variance between means of groups}}{\text{variance within the groups}}$$

and F[1] is then evaluated in Appendix III to obtain the probability that the different groups derive from a single population.

In Figure 10, the means of the four samples shown are quite close to each other, with a variability much less than that within each group, suggesting a possible derivation from one overall population. By contrast, in Figure 11 sample C has a mean far away from the other samples, resulting in a variance of the mean far exceeding the average variance within means. In such a case F is quite high indicative of a sample that derives from a separate population.

One may appreciate that the Student's t for two groups in reality represents a special case of the F test for ANOVA. In the t-test we use the actual difference of means (as opposed to their variance). Note that the units of variance are squares of units. In order to deal with that we then have to use a square root of variance in the demoninator (either SD or SEM). It is indeed not a surprise that $F = t^2$ if you check the values under df $= 1$ (i.e. two groups) for the numerator in Appendix III.

TAKE HOME MESSAGES

- A major interest of statistics is to demonstrate whether or not a point or a set of data belongs to the same population as another group **(null hypothesis)**.
- In nominal data a test for a given disease that is positive in the majority

---

[1]Called F after the English statistician, Sir Ronald Fisher (1890–1962), who introduced the analysis of variance

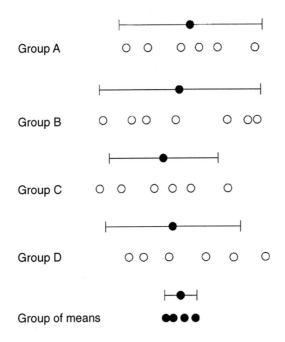

Figure 10   The means of four sample populations are close

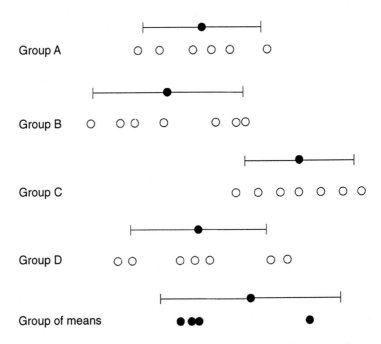

Figure 11   The means of four sample populations are widely separated

of diseased individuals has high **sensitivity**. If a test is negative in the majority of normals, it has **high specificity**.

- Even though sensitivity and specificity are important characteristics of a test, we often have to resort to values such as **predictive value** of a positive or negative test. This is because the prevalence of a disease may play a significant role. For instance, in a rare disease a positive result with even a very sensitive test is more likely to signify a false positive individual rather than the occasional true positive patient.

- In continuous data we use two cut offs to find whether two groups originate from different populations, and thus reject the null hypothesis (i.e. that both are part of one population). α stands for our cut off below which we assume that a value is deviant and thus unlikely to come from that group. An α **of 0.05** (often expressed as $p < 0.05$) is the usual α cut off. β stands for our cut off accepted for overlap of data from the other group for the point that gives on α of 0.05. We usually accept $\beta = 0.2$ (or a **power, $1 - \beta = 0.8$**). Similar to sensitivity and specificity (equivalent to β and α, respectively for continuous data), the moment you decrease α (to be sure that the groups are different) you simultaneously increase β (increase the overlap of the other group).

- One can use an appropriate equation to predict the number of subjects needed for a given research questions when α and β are set.

- In principle, when we try to compare different groups we compare the variability of the means of the groups to that of the data within the groups (analysis of variance, F). When only two groups are present, this simplifies to comparing the difference of the means to the standard error of the mean (Student's t-test – see next Chapter).

QUESTIONS

1. The Captopril scan test has been used as a diagnostic procedure to evaluate the presence of renovascular hypertension (RVH). The test has a sensitivity of 95%, and a specificity of 90%. What percentage of subjects with a positive test will indeed have RVH, if the test is used as a screening procedure in 10 000 unselected hypertensives (RVH prevalence 2%)?

2. What percent of RVH patients will be present in patients with positive Captopril test, if the procedure is performed in 100 young (age 18–25 years) hypertensive females (RVH prevalence 65%)?

3. A new promising medication is found and you would like to evaluate it. You do not want to miss a possible effect. You will:
   (a) Decrease α to less than 0.05,
   (b) Increase power to higher than 0.80,

(c) Both,

(d) Neither.

4. A new antihypertensive drug is on the market. You plan to compare it with the one you presently use. Given the significant rate of complications with the new medication, you would like to be sure that the new one is superior to the conventional treatment. Before you conclude so, you will:

   (a) Decrease α level to less than 0.05,

   (b) Increase power to higher than 0.80,

   (c) Both,

   (d) Neither.

5. You wish to evaluate the effect of a new medication that presumably decreases serum cholesterol. If the level of cholesterol in the group to which you plan to give the drug is 280 ± 20 (mean $\pm$ standard deviation), how many subjects do you need to recruit if:

   (a) You anticipate that the drug will decrease cholesterol by 30 mg/dl and you select $p < 0.05$ and a power of 0.80,

   (b) You select a $p < 0.01$ and a power of 0.90,

   (c) The drug is expected to decrease cholesterol by 60 mg/dl and you aim for a $p < 0.05$ and power $= 0.95$.

CHAPTER 4

Inferential statistics – comparison of groups with outcome in continuous data

---

When the outcome of interest is in the form of continuous data and two or more groups are to be compared, one has to ask three questions, in order to select the appropriate statistical test.

(1) ARE THE DATA FROM PAIRED SUBJECTS?

By that we mean that the same subjects were submitted to two or more treatments. For instance, the weight before and 2 weeks after beginning a new diuretic medication represents such a situation. In that case the outcome of interest, weight, is evaluated before and after a maneuver, the diuretic, in the same individual. This is a situation that in the case of 2 groups requires paired analysis (paired *t*-test). If there are more than two groups (more observations on the same subject) then another test – repeated measure analysis of variance is needed (see below).

Note that paired experiments are, in principle, more robust than unpaired experiments. For example, if each individual taking a diuretic loses 2 kg in 2 weeks then you can feel comfortable that this represents an effect of the diuretic. In contrast, in two random groups, if one receives placebo and the other the diuretic, a 2 kg weight reduction in the diuretic-treated group is less strong evidence of effectiveness of the medication (Figure 12). This is because the variation of weight in each group is larger than 2 kg, so it is unclear whether the difference between the two groups is a real effect of the diuretic or simply a random small difference in mean weight between the two groups. It follows that, when possible, it is better to evaluate a given manipulation in the same subject. If we deal with unmatched data then we perform an unpaired *t*-test for two groups, or analysis of variance in the case of more than two groups.

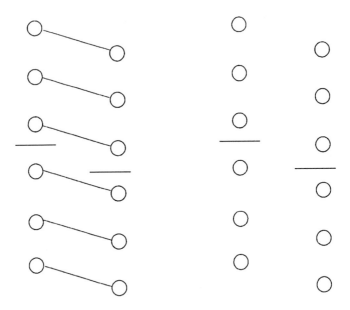

Figure 12 Data are shown from unpaired groups (left panel) and from the same subjects before and after treatment (paired data, right panel). Note that the same means and distribution demonstrates a clear cut effect for the paired data, while no difference is apparent for the unpaired groups

(2) ARE DATA OF EACH GROUP PART OF A NORMAL (BELL-SHAPE) CURVE OR DO THEY CONTAIN DEVIANT POINTS?

Note that Student's[1] *t*-test and analysis of variance are called parametric tests and are used when the continuous data of the outcome (parameter) are part of a normally distributed group. However, if there is substantial variation and the curve is profoundly skewed, one may need to use non-parametric tests. Non-parametric tests should also be used if the data are meaningful in terms of rank but not with regard to actual differences. For instance, let us consider the case where a disease progresses from mild to severe, or from stage I to stage III. Even if we assign numerical values to these situations (for instance APACHE II, a scoring system used to predict mortality in intensive care unit patients), it is clear that a change from mild to moderate is not identical to that from moderate to severe. Under those conditions, it may not be meaningful to use parametric statistics. Instead, use of a non-parametric test is in order.

---

[1]Student in the pseudonym of William Gossett who described it in 1908. He was working for the Guinness Brewery, and was evaluating the different procedures related to beer making. To keep his anonymity and deceive the company's competitors, he published under the pseudonym

Table 10   Weight before and after treatment with diuretics

Subject	Weight (Baseline)	Weight (Diuretic)	Difference	
1	86	84	2	
2	79	77	2	
3	72	68.5	3.5	
4	96	92	4	
5	85	84	1	
6	82	82.5	−0.5	
7	63	61	2	
8	61	59.5	1.5	
9	66	63.5	2.5	
10	69	68	1	
11	73	70.5	2.5	
12	77	75	2	
Mean	75.75	73.79	2.04	
SD	9.97	9.89	0.97	
SEM	2.88	2.85	0.28	$t = 6.08$

(3)   ARE THERE MORE THAN TWO GROUPS TO BE COMPARED?

If we are dealing with two groups, the paired (matched) or unpaired (unmatched) Student's *t*-test is used. If it is necessary to use non-parametric statistics and there are two groups, then the Wilcoxon-signed rank or Mann–Whitney U test is appropriate (see Chapter 6). If there are more than two groups to compare, one has to resort to analysis of variance for parametric statistics and to Friedman or Kruskall–Wallis for non-parametric comparison (see Chapter 6).

Matched groups

In the following pages we will deal with the specific tests. First let us discuss matched data, for example the decrease of body weight (in kg) following the use of an experimental diuretic agent. In Table 10, one appreciates the weight before and after the use of the diuretic in 12 subjects. The difference in weight is identified separately and the mean difference and its standard error of the mean are determined. One can then proceed to determine the:

$$t = \frac{\text{mean } \Delta}{\text{SEM}}$$

and identify in Appendix II, under degrees of freedom, $n - 1$, ($12 - 1 = 11$) the possibility that this difference occurred by chance. For $t = 6.08$, the probability that this difference is random is very small, $p < 0.001$. We

41

Table 11 Systolic blood pressure in patients with hepatic failure and control subjects. Comparison of unpaired groups

	Systolic blood pressure	
	Hepatic failure ($n = 12$)	*Control* ($n = 8$)
	111	133
	116	140
	115	132
	100	129
	121	136
	105	121
	114	125
	103	124
	106	
	113	
	104	
	109	
Mean	109.75	130.00
Standard deviation	6.01	6.0

$$\text{Pooled } \sigma^2 = \frac{(11 \times 6.01^2) + (7 \times 6.04^2) = 36.26}{18}$$

$$\text{Standard error of mean} = \sqrt{[36.26/12]+[36.26/8]} = 2.75$$

$$t = \frac{130 - 109.75}{2.75} = 7.37, \; p < 0.001$$

thus conclude that the difference is real and we present the data as: 75.75 ± 2.88 versus 73.99 ± 2.85, $n = 12$, $p < 0.001$. An alternative way would be to find the 95% confidence limits of the difference as equal to $\Delta \pm t_{n-1}$ SEM. In such case this equals 2.04 ± (2.2 × 0.28): the actual difference is between 1.44 and 2.64. The possibility that there is no actual difference between the two groups, or that mean Δ equals zero is not included in the 95% confidence range; a less than 5% chance of being real. One would then reject this hypothesis, and again conclude that the two groups are indeed different, i.e. that the diuretic has a real effect – to decrease body weight.

Unmatched groups

Let us now move to the comparison of two groups that are not matched, say normal individuals and patients with liver disease (Table 11). Assume that the two groups are age- and sex-controlled, and we evaluate their systolic blood pressures. Again we will attempt to find the *t* value from $t = \dfrac{\text{Difference of mean}}{\text{SEM}}$. The SEM is much more complex because it reflects the different variability (variance) of the two groups, and the different number of subjects that each group contains. A mean variance (σ^2) is calculated from:

$$\sigma^2 = \frac{(n_1 - 1) \cdot \sigma_1^2 + (n_2 - 1) \cdot \sigma_2^2}{(n_1 - 1) + (n_2 - 1)}$$

n_1, n_2, the number of subjects in groups 1 and 2, σ_1, σ_2 the standard deviation of these groups.

and $\quad \text{SEM} = \sqrt{\sigma^2/n_1 + \sigma^2/n_2}$

The *t* value is then determined from the difference of the means of the two groups divided by the SEM determined as described above. As shown in Table 11, *t* = 7.37 indicative of a real difference between the two groups.

More than two groups

As mentioned in Chapter 3, when we deal with more than two groups, we then resort to some form of analysis of variance. In short, we evaluate the variance of the means of the groups relative to the variance of the data within the groups. Their ratio is *F*, and evaluation of *F* in Appendix III allows one to see whether all the groups are likely to be part of a single population, as opposed to groups derived from a different populations.

Unmatched groups

To evaluate more than two groups one has to determine the variance of the means of the groups and compare it to the variance of the data within the groups. Their ratio will be *F*. Before we make our final calculation we have to determine:

(a) the mean ($\bar{x}_i$) and standard deviation (s_i) of each group,
(b) the mean of the means of the groups ($\bar{x}_m$) and their standard deviation (s_m)
(c) the overall mean ($\bar{x}$) and standard deviation (s).

Let us consider three groups of pregnant women, normal first pregnancy, normal subsequent pregnancy and pre-eclamptic, and evaluate their serum uric acid levels (Table 12). The first step is to determine the sum of squares, a result analogous to the sum of the squared differences of the different data from the mean, we used for the Students *t*-test. As

Table 12 Comparison of levels of serum uric acid in three groups of pregnant women

	Serum uric acid (mg/dl)		
	Normal pregnancies		*Pre-eclamptic*
	First Pregnancy	*Multiple Pregnancies*	
	2.3	3.3	5.6
	4.6	5.0	6.8
	3.7	2.6	8.0
	5.1	2.7	7.3
	3.6	4.2	9.0
	4.0	3.6	7.3
	2.9	3.5	6.7
	3.2	4.1	6.6
	3.3	4.0	6.2
$\bar{x}_I$	3.63	3.67	7.06
s_i	0.81	0.71	0.95

$\bar{x} = 4.79$ $s = 1.87$
$\bar{x}_m = 4.79$ $s_m = 1.97$

mentioned above, when we deal with multiple groups, we have to determine separately the differences that derive from variability between the groups, and that that represents variability of the data within the groups.

The sum of squares for the between-groups equals the number of subjects in each group (n) multiplied by the number of the groups minus one ($k - 1$), and then multipled by s_m^2. For the within-groups category, we multiply the number of subjects within each group minus one ($n_i - 1$) by the sum of the variances of each group ($s_1^2 + ... + s_i^2$). Then the variance (mean square) of the data within the groups and the variance of the means of the groups are calculated by dividing the sum of squares by the degrees of freedom ($n - k$, within the groups, and $k - 1$ between the groups). We then divide the variance between groups by the variance within groups (F). We evaluate F in Appendix III against the appropriate degrees of freedom (See Table 13 for calculations).

Stated differently, in ANOVA we subdivide the total variation (SS total) into two parts: that due to deviation of the mean from the grand mean (SS between groups), and that due to deviation of data points from the mean of their group (SS within groups, or residual).

Matched groups

Consider ten subjects treated with antihypertensive A, placebo, and

Table 13 Comparison of levels of serum uric acid in three groups of pregnant women, using analysis of variance (ANOVA)

	Sum of squares *(SS)*	*Degrees of* *freedom*	*Variance* *(mean square, MS)*	*F*
Within groups	$(n_i - 1)(s_1^2 + s_2^2 + ... + s_i^2)*$ $8(0.66 + 0.50 + 0.90) = 16.48$	$n - k$ $27 - 3 = 24$	$MSW = SSW/n - k$ 0.69	
Between groups	$n(k - 1)s_m^2$ $9 \times 2 \times 3.88 = 69.84$	$k - 1$ $3 - 1 = 2$	$MSB = SSB/k - 1$ 34.92	$MSB/MSW =$ 50.61
Total	$(n - 1)s^2$ $26 \times 3.28 = 85.28$	$nk - 1$ $27 - 1 = 26$	3.28	

Stated differently, in ANOVA we subdivide the total variation (SS total) into two parts: that due to deviation of the mean from the grand mean (SS between groups), and that due to deviation of data points from the mean of their group (SS within groups, or residual).

Table 14 Comparison of the effect of two different antihypertensives on the diastolic blood pressure of 12 hypertensives

		Diastolic Blood Pressure					
Subject	*Baseline*	*Drug A*	*Placebo*	*Drug B*	X_{s1}	S_s	S_{ss}^2
1	102	96	100	94	98.0	3.16	10
2	97	92	98	91	94.5	3.04	9.25
3	103	97	101	96	99.25	2.86	8.19
4	112	106	111	107	109.0	2.55	6.00
5	108	105	109	107	107.25	1.48	2.19
6	107	100	107	102	104.0	3.08	9.50
7	106	99	108	100	103.25	3.83	14.69
8	111	97	110	99	104.25	6.30	39.69
9	100	93	98	91	95.5	3.64	13.25
10	99	94	98	89	95.0	3.33	15.50
Mean	104.5	97.9	104.0	97.6	$\Sigma S_s^2 = 128.75$		
SD	4.84	4.48	5.18	6.17			

Total Mean	101.00	X_s	101.01	X_m	101.00	
SD		6.14	S_s	4.98	S_m	3.26

antihypertensive B in sequential fashion (Table 14). One must calculate the following parameters:

(a) The mean of all data ($\bar{x}$) and their standard deviation (s);

(b) The mean of each treatment group (x_m), and the standard deviation of these means (S_m);

(c) The mean of each subject (x_s), standard deviation (s_s) and the sum of s_s^2 (ΣS_s^2).

We first identify the sum of the squares (SS), that is the sum of the differences from the mean squared. We then divide SS by the degrees of

Table 15 Comparison of the effect of two different antihypertensives on the diastolic blood pressure of 12 hypertensives. Use of repeated measures analysis of variance

	SS	Degrees of freedom	Variance or mean square (MS/df)	$F = \dfrac{MS\ effect}{MS\ interaction}$
Subjects	$k(n-1)\,S_s^2$ $4 \times 9 \times 4.98^2 = 892.81$	$n-1$ $10-1=9$	99.20	$10.35,\ p < 0.001$
Techniques	$n\,(k-1)\,S_m^2$ $10 \times 3 \times 3.25^2 = 318.83$	$k-1$ $4-1=3$	106.28	$11.09,\ p < 0.001$
Interactions	total – subject – technology = 258.64	$(n-1)(k-1)$ $9 \times 3 = 27$	9.58	
Total	$(nk-1)s^2$ $39 \times 6.14^2 = 1470.28$	$nk-1$ $40-1=39$	37.70	

freedom to find the mean square (variance). Finally we find F from the ratio of the variance of the mean of the treatment over a variance of individual data. Although this appears quite involved the actual calculations are nothing more than several arithmetic manipulations as shown in Table 15.

If an F is found that indicates that one or more groups are different from the other, then one could perform a t-like test between the two groups to uncover which of the groups are different. There will be two differences from the usual $t = \dfrac{\text{difference}}{\text{SEM}}$.

First, SEM will not be determined in the usual way from the data of the two groups of interest. Instead, SEM will be calculated from the square root of the variance (MS) divided by the number of subjects and will be used for the comparison of any two groups. The second difference will be the so-called Bonferroni modification. You may remember that we said that if the possibility is less than 5% ($p < 0.05$) that two groups make up part of one group, then they are considered different. Note, however, that we have accepted a chance of 1 in 20 (5%) that we may have arrived at the wrong conclusion just by bad 'luck' (α error). An error is more likely to occur if we do more than one comparison. To correct for that, α is adjusted to $\alpha/k(k-1)$, where k = number of groups. Thus for k = 3 groups, decrease by 6, i.e. a $p = 0.05$ will be equal to $p < 0.01$. However, as the number of groups increase, the adjusted α becomes exceedingly small, and a real difference is difficult to identify.

Alternatively, one may elect to use a number of modified t-tests called q tests. Their generic type is:

$$q = \frac{\Delta \text{ means}}{\sqrt{\text{mean square within groups}/n}}$$

Appendix IV shows the q value for this so-called Tukey procedure used for analysis of differences among groups.

A similar test is the Newman–Keuls procedure. This is essentially identical to Tukey but, instead of allowing any comparison, it drives the researcher to go on in a stepwise fashion until no more significant results are found. Since fewer tests are often performed with Newman–Keuls, statistical significance may be easier to be found than with the Tukey test. The q values for Newman–Keuls are shown in Appendix V.

Yet another q test is Dunn's test (Appendix VI). This is not to say that we have exhausted all possible comparison techniques! Scheffe's and Durnett's procedures represent two more. However, it is beyond the scope of this textbook to go into further detail.

TWO-WAY ANOVA

This is a technique that allows us to find out whether a given effect of a treatment holds true for different groups (no interaction) or whether the results differ between the two groups (multiplicative – with interaction). Let us assume that we evaluate the effectiveness of calcium blockers on the cardiac output of patients with systolic and diastolic dysfunction. It is likely that the effects of calcium blockers on cardiac output may be different in the two forms of cardiac failure. The calculations are very tedious and involved and thus far exceed the needs of the usual biostatistical primer.

RANDOMIZED BLOCK DESIGNS

In a sense this represents a modification of ANOVA in which we subdivide the groups and thus 'control' for differences in genetics, age, sex and so forth.

TAKE HOME MESSAGES

- The means of different groups are compared using **analysis of variance**. The presence of an actually different group is suggested when the variability of the means is higher than the variability of the data within the different groups.
- The ratio of the variabilities is called F

$$F = \frac{\text{variance between groups (means)}}{\text{variance within group}}$$

The higher the F, the more one is convinced that at least one group is different.

- If only two groups are to be compared, analysis of variance is somewhat simplified. In that case the difference of the two groups is compared to the variability within the groups (standard error of mean). Their ratio is called t ($t = \frac{\Delta \text{ means}}{\text{SEM}}$) and the test is called **Student's *t*-test**.
- The higher the *t* value, the more one is convinced that the two groups originate from different populations (are different).
- *t* represents a measure of variability of means, more or less like *z* which is a measure of variability of data points around their mean. For an increasing number of data points, *t* approaches *z*, which confirms their similar derivations.
- By rearranging above the equation, one can arrive at the: **confidence limits = Δ mean $\pm\, t$ SEM**.
- If the confidence limits do not contain 0 then one may conclude that the possibility that the groups may come from the same population (where Δ mean = 0) is unlikely.

QUESTIONS

1. Two groups of patients ($n = 25$ in each group) have nephrotic syndrome. Two separate regimens are used for treatment, one in each group. The 24-h urine protein averages 3 g in the first group, and 2 g in the second group. If the overall standard deviation is 2 g, can one say that the regimen used in the second group is better than the one used in the first one?
2. What if each group in question 1 had 100 subjects each, instead of 25?
3. What if the two groups had 3 and 1 g of protein, respectively, 25 subjects each, and again a standard deviation of 2?
4. What if you encounter two groups, each having 4 patients, and 24 h protein of 5 and 2 g respectively, while standard deviation is again 2 g?
5. You have the data of triceps skinfold, a measure of body fat, of three different groups:

normal adult males	normal adult females	adult females with metastatic cancer
10	20	9
8	26	17
15	22	15
13	18	13
12	20	11
7	19	10

Are these groups different with regard to their triceps skinfold?

CHAPTER 5

Inferential statistics –
correlation of continuous data
and linear regression

In the previous chapter we dealt with comparison of groups containing continuous data. However, sometimes our interest centers on how continuous data are affected by a given property which is also expressed as continuous data. In such cases, both the outcome (dependent variable) and the input (independent variable) are continuous data (as shown in the example in Table 16). Statistical techniques such as **linear regression** are needed to deal with such a relationship. We actually encounter many such correlations in real life and in biology. For instance, it is common that rich people (subjects with higher income) buy expensive houses or cars. There thus appears to be a strong relationship to the outcome dependent variable (cost of house in dollars) with the independent variable (income in dollars). Note, however, that the relationship is not always causal, that is the independent variable may not be directly related to the outcome. For example, it is also true that rich people have the highest electric bills. However, the latter may have to do more with their life styles rather than directly with their income. It is understood that if a tycoon were to live in a small studio apartment, he might not use more electricity than the normal-income tenant of such a place.

In medicine, correlation is often noted and may have significant links to understanding of epidemiology and pathophysiology. The relationship of aging (years) to glomerular filtration rate, red blood cell count to sedimentation rate, ejection fraction to cardiac output, cigarette pack-years to expiratory flow rates and so forth are some such examples.

One way to evaluate such a relationship is to plot the data points so that each point has a certain value in both axes: the independent horizontal x axis, and the dependent vertical y axis. One could then divide the data into four quarters. As in Figure 13A or B, if most of the points fall in the two diagonally opposite quarters then one may feel comfortable that a real relationship among the two data sets exists. If, on the other hand, all quarters have a similar number of data, it is likely that the two parameters do not relate to each other (Figure 13C).

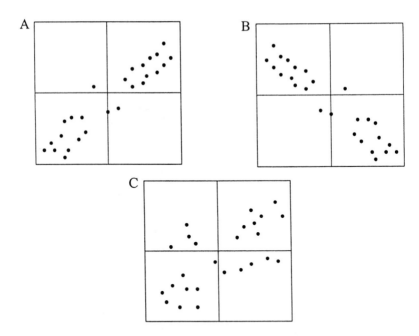

Figure 13 Schematic representation of different correlations. Panel A demonstrates a tight direct relation. Panel B depicts a tight, but inverse correlation. In both panels, the bulk of the data fall in the two diagonally opposed quarters. In panel C data appear in all quarters, evidence of poor or no significant correlation

Of course, when dealing with data, we need a more quantitative way to find out if such a relationship exists, rather than the qualitative (optical) way just described. Similar to what was said in the previous Chapters, we need to test the null hypothesis. In the case of correlation, we hypothesize that any trend for a relationship is accidental and that indeed there is no correlation. If this appears unlikely ($p < 0.05$), we then acknowledge that indeed such a relationship exists at a statistically significant level. Essentially, we are examining how much of the variance of the dependent data points is due to (or could be predicted by) change of the independent variable. Since there are a number of different modes of possible correlation, including linear and curvilinear relationships, we must first select the mode of possible correlation. For our present introductory course we will use **linear regression**[1].

In linear regression there are two steps to deal with. First, we have to construct the best posssible line that can express the relationship of the

[1]The term regression was introduced by anthropologist Sir Francis Galton to explain the relationship in height between fathers and sons

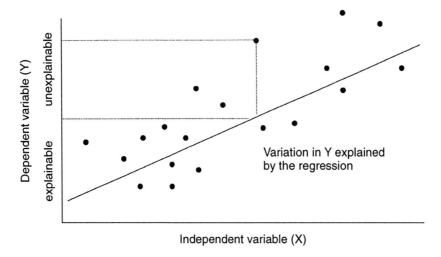

Figure 14 Schematic representation of the extent that a linear regression explains the dependent variable y

two parameters. Then we have to examine the extent to which the relationship can account for the data distribution.

Let us start with the line that best fits the data. The best fit will be obtained when the sum of distances of the different points (or their squares) from the regression line will be the smallest possible. The equation that describes the relation of y to x is: y = a + bx. In this equation, **a** represents the starting point or **intercept**, and **b** the **slope**. It is understood that the data points will not always fall in the line described by the equation. The distance of a point from the line represents what remains unexplained by the linear regression (Figure 14). The line that best describes the relatioship of y to x shall have the smallest possible sum of the squares of the distance of the different points from the line (**least squares**).

Once the line is constructed, we then identify how much of the variance of a given point is due to the effect of this least square line (Figure 15). All points have both a y and an x value. One can approach a given y value as part of an overall y population in a similar way to that previously shown for continuous data. Thus there will be a mean y value ($\bar{y}$) and a spread around the mean. The fact that points move in more than one dimension (i.e. up and down) suggests that they are **not only** affected by the distribution on the y axis (up and down) **but also** by their x value (x axis, left to right). This correlation between x and y is represented by the line produced by the least squares. A point (y_i) that lies on the line could be said to vary from its expected mean ($\bar{y}$) exclusively because of the

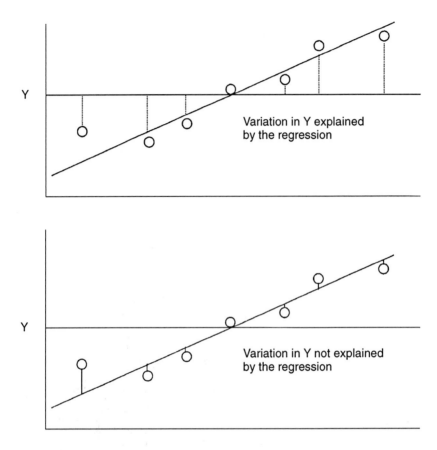

Figure 15   Top panel shows the extent that the variation of the dependable variable y is explained by the linear regression. Bottom panel depicts the extent that the variability of y is not explained

correlation. Alternatively, the correlation could account exclusively for the movement of this point away from the mean. In terms of mathematical formulations, one could separate variance into two components. First, the variance of each dependent point y from its mean y and each point x from its mean similar to that previously described, i.e.

$$\text{variance } y = \frac{\Sigma(y-\bar{y})^2}{n} \qquad \text{Similarly variance } x = \frac{\Sigma(x-\bar{x})^2}{n}$$

The variability due to correlation can be found from the difference of a given point from both the mean of the dependent data $\bar{y}$ and its difference from that of the mean of the independent data, x, so that:

$$\text{variance}_{x,y} = \frac{\Sigma(x-\bar{x})(y-\bar{y})}{n}$$

The proportion of variance due to the regression (r^2) will then equal:

$$r^2 = \frac{(\text{variance}_{x,y}) \cdot (\text{variance}_{x,y})}{(\text{variance } x) \cdot (\text{variance } y)}$$

$$r^2 = \frac{\Sigma(x-\bar{x})(y-\bar{y})/n \cdot \Sigma(x-x)(y-\bar{y})/n}{\Sigma(y-\bar{y})^2/n \cdot \Sigma(x-\bar{x})^2/n}$$

or $$r^2 = \frac{\left[\Sigma(x-\bar{x})(y-\bar{y})\right]^2}{\Sigma(y-\bar{y})^2 \cdot \Sigma(x-\bar{x})^2}$$

There are two points worth noting. First, r^2 could have a value ranging between 0 and 1. One shows that all the points lie on the line, so that the line accounts for 100% of the data. In contrast, an r^2 value of 0 indicates complete lack of correlation. An r^2 value of 0.6 suggest that linear regression is responsible for 60% of the point's variation, or that 60% of the data could be explained by it. Note than in most of the literature you will encounter r as opposed to r^2. This is simply the square root of r^2, has a higher value (square root is higher for numbers between 0 and 1) and therefore looks more impressive! An added advantage is that most tables that show the significance of a correlation are constructed for r. As shown in Appendix VII, if r is determined, one may find the level of significance of a linear regression. Irrespective of statistical significance, always be suspect of an $r < 0.3$ because this is equal to an $r^2 < 0.1$, i.e. the regression accounts for less than 10% of data distribution.

This brings us to the second point. In the sum of squares we have encountered so far, the value has always been positive. This is because we square the difference from the mean and thus even a negative difference becomes positive. This may not be true with linear regression. Since each point has two differences $(x-\bar{x})$ and $(y-\bar{y})$, they are multiplied by each other, rather than by themselves. In such a case, the variance and r may have a negative sign. A negative sign indicates that as one parameter increases, the other decreases. Thus, a negative r suggest that the relationship is inverse (negative linear regression).

Let us complete the issue of linear regression by determining the slope of the least square line. This can be computed from the variance of the regression relative to the variance of the independent variable x, i.e.

$$\text{slope B} = \frac{\Sigma(x-\bar{x})(y-\bar{y})}{\Sigma(x-\bar{x})^2}$$

The intercept point on the y axis can then be calculated by plotting b and the mean $\bar{x}$ and $\bar{y}$ in the slope equation that $\bar{y} = a + bx$ and solving for a.

Table 16 Linear regression between height and weight in 10 men

Height (cm) x	Weight (kg) y	$(x - \bar{x})$	$(x - \bar{x})^2$	$(y - \bar{y})$	$(y - \bar{y})^2$	$(x - \bar{x}) \cdot (y - \bar{y})$
170	70	−4	16	−3.9	15.21	15.60
165	64	−9	81	−9.9	98.01	89.10
180	81	6	36	7.1	50.41	42.60
186	85	12	144	11.1	123.21	133.20
179	77	5	25	3.1	9.61	15.50
175	75	1	1	1.1	1.21	1.1
163	64	−11	121	−9.9	98.01	108.90
169	70	−5	25	−3.9	15.21	19.50
171	72	−3	9	−1.9	3.61	5.70
182	81	8	72	7.1	50.41	56.80
Sum 1740	739	0	530	0	464.90	488.00
Mean 174	73.9					

regression equation: y (weight) = −86.31 + (0.92 × height)

$$b = \frac{\sum(x - \bar{x})(y - \bar{y})}{\sum(x - \bar{x})^2} = \frac{488}{530} = 0.92 \qquad a = \bar{y} - b\bar{x} = 73.9 - (0.92 \times 174) = -86.81$$

$$r^2 = \frac{\left[\sum(x - \bar{x})(y - \bar{y})\right]^2}{\sum(x - \bar{x})^2 \cdot \sum(y - \bar{y})^2} = \frac{(488)^2}{530 \times 464.90} = 0.97 \qquad r = \sqrt{r^2} = \sqrt{0.97} = 0.98$$

Table 16 shows an example of a linear regression between height and weight in ten men.

Although solving a linear regression appears (and indeed is) a tedious process, most modern calculators and all statistical computer programs make this easy. The only reason we have gone through the way to calculate this manually is to clarify the way one constructs a line, the meaning of *r* and *r²*, and how significance is identified.

It should be mentioned that frequently more than one factor can influence the value of the dependent variable. For instance, erythrocyte sedimentation rate is influenced by both the number of red cells and the ratio of albumin to globulin. In that case, both parameters are acting independently of each other. On the other hand, the level of pCO_2 in the blood of patients with chronic obstructive pulmonary disease relates both to mid-expiratory flow rate and the 1 second forced vital capacity (FEV1). However, since these two tests are inter-related (they both reflect the same pathophysiologic mechanisms), having both tests does not further enhance the tightness of the relationship produced by either of these parameters individually.

It is certainly beyond the scope of this textbook to describe in any detail the use of **multiple linear regression** to assess the relationship of multiple variables to a given dependent factor. Most statistical computer programs will perform these tedious calculations in just a few minutes. Nonetheless, it is important to identify the pertinent points relevant to understanding the processes one has to go through. One approach is to identify the relationship of each parameter to the dependent variable and identify the r^2 for each one separately. Then keep adding one parameter at a time for as long as the combination's r^2 rises to a level higher than the previous combination. We proceed this way until further additions show no further effect. One may elect to go the other way around: identify an equation with all parameters included. Then try to eliminate each parameter separately, if removal of one factor appears to have no effect on r^2, then this factor is eliminated as independently unimportant. In contrast, if the lack of a factor produces a significant decrease in r^2 then this factor has a significant role in determining the dependent parameter and thus stays in the final equation. One proceeds until all remaining factors are significant.

TAKE HOME MESSAGE

- **Linear regression** describes the correlation among two or more (multiple) continuous data sets;
- r^2 describes the proportion of the independent variable(s) that is/ are responsible (account) for the linear relationship;
- r^2 ranges between 0 (no relationship) and 1 (perfect relationship). Intermediate values indicate that the linear regression accounts for a percentage of the variation of the data. (i.e. an r^2 of 0.6 indicates the linear regression accounts for 60% of the variation);
- r ranges between –1 and +1. Negative values describe an inverse relationship, while positive values indicate a direct relationship. Zero stands for no relationship while either –1 or 1 suggest a perfect relationship. Intermediate values indicate an in-between, though not exact, situation.

QUESTIONS ·

1. 16 normal adult men have their body weight and 24-h urine creatinine determined. Both parameters are influenced by the size of muscles. A positive linear regression is found: 24-h creatinine (mg) = 22 × body weight (kg) + 50, $r = 0.7$
   (a) Is this a significant relationship?
   (b) Does it mean that 70% of the values of creatinine are controled by the body weight?
   (c) Does it prove that creatinine production (and thus excretion) is controlled by the body weight?
2. What if, in the example above (question #1), they were 10 normal adult males instead of 16?

3. r^2 is:
   (a) A measure of the variability of the slope.
   (b) A characteristc of the regression that ranges between −1 to +1.
   (c) A reflection of the proportion of the independent variable that is predicted by the dependent variable.
4. A linear regression is found for 150 subjects with $r = 0.3$ and $p < 0.001$. How will you describe this relationship?
5. A tight linear regression is found for 24-h urinary creatinine versus either height ($r = 0.81$), or weight ($r = 0.79$). However no further improvement is found when a multiple linear regression is attempted ($r = 0.83$). How do you explain it?

CHAPTER 6

Inferential statistics:
non-parametric – ordinal data

So far we have dealt with continuous data (parametric techniques). Implicit in them was that the data were distributed normally. However, this is not always the case. This is particularly significant when we deal with obvious non-normally distributed data in a small data set (< 50 subjects). In those situations it is much better to rank the data and compare the rank of one group relative to that of the other. In this way we will avoid the error that would be introduced by including the values of outliers.

It should be noted that we are sometimes forced to use ranked (ordinal) data when it has values that do not have continuous variability. This is particularly true when we deal with arbitary scores such as disease stages (stage I, II, III, IV) where the difference in stages does not signify a numerical difference. The case is similar with arbitary scores, such as Glasgow score for coma, APGAR for neonates, or APACHE scoring for patients in intensive care.

Most of the tests used for ordinal data are much simpler to perform arithmetically. In fact, most have been developed as quick and easy methods of bypassing the often tedious calculations encountered in the parametric techniques described in the previous chapters. It is of interest that, although these tests are not as robust as the parametric techniques, they are almost as efficient as the former in detecting differences, even when used for data where a normal distribution is satisfied.

Two major differences exist between parametric and ordinal tests. First, in ordinal tests we compare medians and ranks rather than means and standard deviation. Second, we cannot derive confidence intervals (actually we could but it is a complex and tedious job). With the widespread availability of calculators and computers, their intrinsic ease is not as appealing. The different ordinal tests used and their parametric equivalent are shown in Table 17. In the subsequent few paragraphs we will describe the three most commonly used tests, the Wilcoxon signed rank test, the Wilcoxon rank sum test (also called the Mann-Whitney U-test) and the Spearman rank correlation.

Table 17 Comparison of ordinal and parametric tests

Ordinal test	Parametric equivalent
Wilcoxon signed rank test	Paired Student *t*-test
Wilcoxon rank sum test Mann–Whitney U test Kendal S test	Student *t*-test
Kruskal–Wallis test	One way analysis of variance (ANOVA)
Friedman test	Repeated measures ANOVA
Spearman rank correlation Kendal rank correlation	Linear regression correlation

WILCOXON SIGNED RANK TEST

You may remember that in Chapter 4 we used the paired *t*-test, a parametric technique, to evaluate the differences in weight in subjects before and after the use of diuretics (Table 10). We could test the same data with ordinal techniques by using the Wilcoxon signed rank test. In such a case, we evaluate the relative magnitude of the differences and their signs rather than their values. Table 18 shows the data calculated in both ways. In Wilcoxon signed rank the difference between the paired values are recorded and the absolute differences are ranked. If more than one difference has the same value then the average rank is used. The ranks are then given a positive or negative sign based on their original difference. The sum of the positive ranks is calculated and is compared to the sum of negative ranks. If it is significantly different, the possibility of a genuine difference is suggested. One may then take the smallest of T+ and T− and apply to Appendix VIII to evaluate the significance. In our case T+ is 1 which shows that the probability of the two groups to be similar is very low, $p \ll 0.01$.

MANN–WHITNEY U TEST (WILCOXON RANK SUM TEST)

When we compared two groups in parametric statistics, we used the Student *t*-test (Table 11). Let us consider again the systolic blood pressure data in the same two groups. To evaluate these two groups in a non-parametric way, the different systolic pressures can be ranked from 1 to 20 (Table 19). If two or more values are identical they get the same rank which will be averaged. For instance blood pressure of 121 is found twice and so each is given a rank of 12.5, since rank 12 and 13 would have been the subsequent two ranks. Of course the next value will get the next rank available, that is 14. If three values had been 121 then each will have been

Table 18 Weight, before and after diuretic treatment. Paired analysis is performed using both parametric (Student *t*-test) and non-parametric (Wilcoxon signed rank test) techniques.

Subject	Parametric paired t-test			Ordinal Wilcoxon signed rank		
	Weight (baseline)	Weight (diuretic)	Difference	Absolute difference	Rank	Signed
1	86	84	2	2	6	6
2	79	77	3	3	10	10
3	72	68.5	3.5	3.5	11	11
4	96	92	4	4	12	12
5	85	84	1	1	2.5	2.5
6	82	82.5	−0.5	0.5	1	−1
7	63	61	2	2	6	6
8	61	59.5	1.5	1.5	4	4
9	66	63.5	2.5	2.5	8.5	8.5
10	69	68	1	1	2.5	2.5
11	73	70.5	2.5	2.5	8.5	8.5
12	77	75	2	2	6	6
Mean	75.75	73.79	2.04	$T+ = 76$		
Standard deviation	9.89	9.89	1.16	$T- = 1$		
Standard error of mean	2.88	2.85	0.34	$t = 6.08$		

assigned a rank 13 (the average of 12,13,14) and so on. U is then calculated from

$$U = (n_1 \cdot n_2) + \frac{n_1\,(n_1 + 1)}{2} - R_1 = (12 \times 8) + \frac{12(12 + 1)}{2} - 78.5 = 95.5$$

where R_1 is the sum of the ranks of one of the groups. One should also find the U for the remaining group, and select the largest value.

This technique is called the Mann–Whitney U test and the values of U are used in Appendix IX to evaluate the probability that the two groups originate from the same population. In view of the fact that such possibility is small $(p < 0.05)$, we conclude once more that the two groups are dissimilar. In other words, patients with liver disease have a lower blood pressure than controls.

THE KRUSKAL–WALLIS TEST

This is the non-parametric equivalent of ANOVA. Similar to all non-parametric techniques, all data are transformed to ranks. If we know the sum of ranks of each group (R_i),the number of the observations in each

Table 19 Systolic blood pressure in patients with hepatic failure and normal control subjects. Comparison is performed by using both parametric, and non-parametric techniques

	Systolic blood pressure		Rank	
	Hepatic failure (n = 12)	Control (n = 8)	Hepatic failure	Control
	111	133	7	18
	116	140	11	20
	115	132	10	17
	100	129	1	16
	121	136	12.5	19
	105	121	4	12.5
	114	125	9	15
	103	124	2	14
	106		5	
	113		8	
	104		3	
	109		6	
Mean	109.75	130	Total 78.5	
Standard deviation (s)	6.01	6.04		

Pooled $S^2 = \dfrac{(11 \times 6.01^2) + (7 \times 6.04^2)}{18} = 36.26$

Standard error of mean $= \sqrt{36.26/12 + 36/26/8} = 2.75$

$t = \dfrac{130 - 109.75}{2.75} = 7.37, \ p < 0.001$

group (n_i), and the number of all observations in the study (N), then one will be able to calculate H, and from that, to evaluate the likelihood of a real difference between the groups. If each group has 5 or more subjects one may evaluate the significance, using chi-square instead of H (see Chapter 7) and number of group (k) minus 1 degrees of freedom (Appendix XI). The data already shown in Table 12 are presented again in Table 20, this time in the form of ranks. The calculations needed to identify H are shown immediately after.

The best test to compare the different groups, is the Dunn procedure. For that, we divide the sum of ranks of the groups we are interested in by the number of subjects in these groups, and thus we derive the mean rank for each group. Then we identify the standard error of mean of the two groups: SEM $= \sqrt{N(N+1)(1/n_1 + 1/n_1)/12}$. Dunn's Q is then

Table 20 Serum uric acid levels for three group of pregnant women. Statistical analysis is performed using non-parametric (Kruskal–Wallis) techniques

First pregnancy	Rank	Serum uric acid (mg/dl) Multiple pregnancies	Rank	Pre-eclamptic	Rank
2.3	1	3.3	6.5	5.6	19
4.6	16	5.0	17	6.8	23
3.7	11	2.6	2	8.0	26
5.1	18	2.7	3	7.3	24.5
3.6	9.5	4.2	15	9.0	27
4.0	12.5	3.6	9.5	7.3	24.5
2.9	4	3.5	8	6.7	22
3.2	5	4.1	14	6.6	21
3.3	6.5	4.0	12.5	6.2	20
ΣR_i	83.5		87.5		207

$$H = \left[\frac{12}{N(N+1)} \Sigma R_i^2 / n_i \right] - \left[3 \cdot (N+1) \right]$$

$= [(12/(27 \times 28) \times (83.5^2/9 + 87.5^2/9 + 87.5^2/9 + 207^2/9)] - [3 \times 28] = 17.69$,

which for d.f. = 2, $p < 0.001$

determined from the ratio of the difference of the mean rank by the SEM of the two groups. We then evaluate for significance (Appendix VI). As is the case in Student–Newman–Keuls procedure, we start with comparison of the two groups furthest apart (i.e. the groups with the largest difference of their mean rank), and proceed until we reach two groups with no significant difference. In Appendix V, k stands for the number of groups spanned by the comparisons.

FRIEDMAN TEST

If we deal with a number of treatments on the same subjects we use the Friedman test. This test is quite similar to the Kruskal–Wallis test just described. The major difference is that in Friedman we evaluate directly for χ^2. Another difference is that we rank each treatment on every subject separately. To allow some better understanding, I have provided, in Table 21, the data from Table 14 transformed to ranks and have identified χ^2.

SPEARMAN RANK CORRELATION

Frequently we need to evaluate the relationship of one variable to another. If either or both data (dependent or independent variables) are likely to

Table 21   Data from Table 14 transformed to ranks

Subject	Baseline	Drug A	Placebo	Drug B
1	4	2	3	1
2	3	2	4	1
3	4	2	3	1
4	4	1	3	2
5	3	1	4	2
6	3.5	1	3.5	2
7	3	1	4	2
8	4	1	3	2
9	4	2	3	1
10	4	2	3	1
	36.5	15	33.5	15

$\chi^2 = 12/(k.n)\ (R_i^2/n + \ldots R_i^2/n) - 3\ (k+1)n$

$\chi^2 = 12/(4 \times 10)(36.5^2/10 + 33.5^2/10 + 15^2/10) - 3\ (4+1)\ 10 = 24.27,\ p < 0.001$

be skewed or to be represented by ranks one may have to deal with a non-parametric evaluation of correlation. The data already shown in Table 16 are presented again in Table 22, this time in non-parametric fashion. Each subject is ranked separately with regard to height and weight. The difference of the two ranks is then identified and then squared (d^2). An R for non-parametric correlation, called Spearman rank correlation coefficient, is then identified as follow:

$$R_s = 1 - \frac{6\Sigma d^2}{n(n^2-1)}$$

The significance of this linear regression can be identified in the same way we described for R, by evaluating R_s in Appendix X.

TAKE HOME MESSAGES

- Data are **ranked** in non-parametric statistical analysis.
- **Ranks** of **groups** can be **compared** (**Wilcoxon, Mann–Whitney** for two groups; **Kruskal–Wallis Friedman** for more).
- **Ranks** can be **correlated** (**Spearman correlation**).
- **Ordinal statistics** are less parametric, but still quite powerful.
- **Ordinal** statistics are preferred for:
  - (a) Continuous **data** that are **skewed,**
  - (b) Data represented by an **arbitrary scale** where variation is less well described or subjective.

Table 22 Data from Table 16 transformed into ranks. Spearman correlation is calculated

Subject (rank)	Height (rank)	Weight d	Difference d	d²
1	4	3.5	0.5	0.25
2	2	1.5	0.5	0.25
3	8	8.5	−0.5	0.25
4	10	10	0	0
5	7	7	0	0
6	6	6	0	0
7	1.5	1.5	0	0
8	3.5	3.5	0	0
9	5	5	0	0
10	8.5	8.5	0	0
				Sum 0.75

$$R_s = 1 - \frac{6\Sigma d^2}{n(n^2-1)} = \frac{1-6\times1.5}{10(100-1)} = 0.99$$

$p < 0.001$

QUESTIONS

1. Solve question #5, Chapter 4 using non-parametric techniques.
2. A sample of 10 medical students evaluate their three common instructors in pediatrics. The scale used ranged from 5 for excellent to 1 for less than acceptable. Their scores were:

Student	Instructor 1	Instructor 2	Instructor 3
1	5	5	4
2	4	3	2
3	4	3	3
4	3	3	3
5	5	3	4
6	5	4	5
7	4	3	4
8	4	4	3
9	4	4	3
10	3	3	2

   Is there a difference among these groups?
3. Solve question #5 of Chapter 4 assuming they were only two groups (A and B).
4. Solve question #2 (above) assuming we deal with instructors 1 and 3 only.
5. Is there any significant correlation in the way students judged instructors 1 and 3?

CHAPTER 7

Inferential statistics: non-parametric – nominal data

Sometimes the outcome of an analysis can be described as nominal. For instance, when we evaluate survival (alive or dead), or presence or absence of disease (positive or negative for systemic lupus erythematosus, based on accepted criteria). If we elect to compare two or more groups with nominal outcomes, the intention is to compare the success and failure rate of each group to what would be expected if all the data were from one group. The differences between observed and expected values are squared and divided by the expected value. They are then summed in a way similar to that previously undertaken. The sum of squares in this situation is called χ^2 (chi square) and is evaluated for significance for degrees of freedom equal to $(r-1)(c-1)$ where r and c stand for rows and columns respectively (Appendix XI). Table 23 shows the comparison of 5-year survival of patients with a given malignancy treated in three different ways. The obvious advantage of the χ^2 test is that it can employ as many groups as one may wish, and there is no need for tedious work, such as that required in analysis of variance. Furthermore, comparison of any two groups could be done without the complex modification described in Chapter 4 for continuous data. On the other hand, one should not lose track of the fact that nominal data are not as robust as continuous. It is therefore imperative to use continuous data whenever possible (as described in detail in Chapters 1 and 2).

A very common situation is that of two groups both containing nominal data. In Table 24 you find the 5-year survival of the first two groups from the previous Table. In such cases the data can be formulated in a contingency 2×2 table as shown:

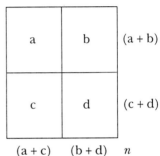

a	b	(a + b)
c	d	(c + d)
(a + c)	(b + d)	n

Table 23 Five-year survival in three different groups of patients provided with different treatments

Groups	Total	Survived (O)	Expected (E)	(O − E)	(O − E)²	(O − E)²/E	Died (O)	Expected (E)	(O − E)	(O − E)²	(O − E)²/E
A	96	53	59.03	−6.03	36.36	0.62	43	36.97	6.03	36.36	0.98
B	111	82	68.25	13.75	189.06	2.77	29	42.75	−13.75	189.06	4.42
C	115	63	70.71	−7.71	59.44	0.84	52	44.29	7.71	59.44	1.34
Total	322	198		0		4.23	124		0		6.74

$\chi^2 = 4.23 + 6.74 = 10.97$, $p < 0.05$

and χ^2 can be calculated from a shortcut formula:

$$\chi^2 = \frac{n\,(ad - bc)^2}{(a + c)\,(b + d)\,(a + b)\,(c + d)}$$

If n is less than 50 it is suggested that the Yates correction be used which modifies the formula to:

$$\chi^2 = \frac{\Sigma\,[(O - E) - 0.5]^2}{E}$$

and the shortcut formula to:

$$\chi^2 = \frac{n\,(ad - bc - 0.5)^2}{(a + c)\,(b + d)\,(a + b)\,(c + d)}$$

Note that if any of the cells has a value less than 5 or n is less than 20 (some suggest even less than 40) it is suggested that the Fisher exact test be used instead, where the probability p is directly determined from:

$$p = \frac{(a + b)!\,(c + d)!\,(a + c)!\,(b + d)!}{a!\;b!\;c!\;d!}$$

A third way to deal with nominal data is to present the two groups as proportions and solve for z, in a way analogous to that method described for continuous data. As stated in Chapter 2, the distribution of data derived from proportion approaches normal distribution as the number of subject (n) increases. The equation used is:

$$Z = \frac{\Delta\ \text{proportions}}{\text{SEM}} = \frac{P_1 - P_2}{\sqrt{P(1 - P)(1 / n_1 + 1 / n_2)}}$$

where p is the average proportion calculated from

$$p\ (\text{proportion}) = \frac{n_1 P_2 + n_2 P_2}{n_1 + n_2}$$

and $\quad \text{SEM}(P_1 - P_2) = \sqrt{\dfrac{P(1 - P)}{n_1} + \dfrac{(P1 - P)}{n_2}} = \sqrt{P(1 - P)(1 / n_1 + 1 / n_2)}$

Note that $z^2 = \chi^2$, so solving for z is just another way to tackle the same problem instead of directly dealing with χ^2.

Yet another (fourth) method exists if one uses the odds ratio (OP) which is equal to: $OR = ad/bc$. In that case a confidence interval is calculated from:

Confidence interval = $OR \times e^{[\pm z\sqrt{(1/a)+(1/b)+(1/c)+(1/d)}\,]}$

which for a 95% interval = $OR \times e^{(\pm 1.96\sqrt{(1/a)+(1/b)+(1/c)+(1/d)})}$

Even though this approach appears very different, it is also, in effect, an indirect product of χ^2 and indeed the 95% confidence limits can become = $OR^{(1\pm 1.96\sqrt{\chi^2})}$ or $OR^{(1\pm 1.96/z)}$.

In the confidence limits we again test the null hypothesis. If the two groups come from the same population,we expect to get a sample with an odds ratio of 1. If 1 is outside the confidence limits we suggest that the groups are different.

A parenthesis is needed here to briefly discuss relative risk and odd ratio. **Relative risk (RR)** is the incidence of disease or positive test in those with a given positive factor (for instance high blood pressure) relative to the incidence in those that lack this factor. Note, that relative risk can only be determined in **prospective studies** when the factor is determined at the onset of the study and the disease or positive test develops in a prespecified period of time. It is calculated as follow:

$$RR = \frac{a/(a+b)}{c/(c+d)}$$

Odds risk or **odds ratio (OR)** is the estimate of relative risk from retrospective (case–control) studies. As already said $OR = \frac{ad}{bc}$, and a 95% confidence limit could be calculated.

In addition to the definitions of OR and RR we have just discused, it is worth dealing with some more parameters that derive from them and are commonly used. If, for instance, the relative risk for a symptom or sign following a treatment is 0.4 (i.e. 40% of the control), this suggests that the risk has decreased by 60%, or that we have a relative risk reduction (RRR) of $1 - RR = 1 - 0.4 = 0.6$. Another parameter of significance is that of the absolute risk reduction (ARR). If, for instance, the usual treatment of a given cancer has a 5-year mortality of 50% and a new surgical procedure reduces that to 20%, then the RRR will be 60%, and the ARR will be –30% (20% – 50%) or 0.3. One of the important attributes of ARR is that its inverse (1/ARR) represents the number of subjects one needs to treat so that one will benefit from the new treatment. In our example $1/0.3 = 3.33$, it suggests that by treating a few more than 3 patients will allow one to survive that would have died if treated with the standard treatment (if we had 4 patients, 2 were expected to have died with the usual therapy and one or less with the new one). As indicated before (end of Chapter 2), these maneuvers together with the modified Bayes' theorem, represent the backbone of the so-called evidence-based medicine, and represent one more line of evidence that statistics have a direct application in biologic research and the practice of medicine.

Table 24   2 × 2 Contingency Tables

(A) **Regular method**

Survived	Expected	$(O-E)^2/E$	Died	Expected	$(O-E)^2/E$
53	59.03	0.62	43	36.97	0.98
82	68.25	2.77	29	42.75	4.42

$\chi^2 = 0.62 + 2.77 + 0.98 + 4.42 = 8.79$
$p < 0.005$

(B) **Short Cut**

	Survived	Died	Total
Group A	53a	43b	96
Group B	82c	29d	111
Total	135	72	207 = N

$$\chi^2 = \frac{n\,(ad-bc)^2}{(a+c)(b+d)(a+b)(c+d)} = \frac{207\,[(53\times29)-(82\times43)]}{135\times72\times96\times111} = 7.91$$

$p < 0.005$

(C) **Proportions**
Group A, $n = 96$ $\qquad$ $P_1 = 53/96 = 0.55$
Group B, $n = 111$ $\qquad$ $P_2 = 82/111 = 0.74$

$$P = \frac{(96\times0.55)+(111\times0.74) = 0.65}{96+111}$$

$$Z = \frac{P_1-P_2}{\sqrt{P(1-P)(1/n_1+1/n_2)}} = 2.88 \qquad Z^2 = 8.28$$

$p < 0.005$

(D) **Odds Ratio**

95% Confidence limits $= \mathrm{OR} \times e^{(\pm1.96\sqrt{(1/a)+(1/b)+(1/c)+(1/d)})}$
OR $= 53\times29/(82\times43) = 0.44$, 95% CI $= 0.44 \times (0.56 \text{ to } 1.79)$
$e^{+1.96...} = 1.79$ $\qquad\qquad = 0.25$ to 0.79
$e^{-1.96....} = 0.56$
$\qquad\qquad$ Also, 95% CI $\quad = \mathrm{OR}^{(1\pm1.96/z)} = \mathrm{OR}\,(1.69 \text{ to } 0.31)$
$\qquad\qquad$ (See text below) $\quad = 0.25$ to 0.78

Table 25 Incidence of headache with/without new medication

		Headache in control individuals	
		Yes	No
Headache in patients	Yes	22	9
taking the medication	No	1	53

$$\chi^2 = \frac{([b-c]-1)^2}{(b+c)} = \frac{49}{10} = 4.9$$

Before we conclude our discussion on comparison of groups based on nominal outcomes, let us now deal with the McNemar χ^2 for paired and matched observations. Let us assume we evaluate the incidence of an event, headache, in the same group when given a new medication or placebo sequentially (Table 25). In this case determination of χ^2 is quite simple since we care only about individuals who showed a variable response (have headache with medication and not with placebo, or vice versa). The logic is quite complex and beyond the scope of this text. However, the calculations are reasonably simple as can be appreciated in Table 25.

It is rather obvious that McNemar is to be used not only for paired observation, as in the previous example described, it can also be used when the effects of a medication, situation or disease on a nominal property is compared against that of its absence in a matched group.

In McNemar we compared two different situations (complications, treatments) in the same subjects. We were able to evaluate whether the two interventions had similar or different effects by using the χ^2 test. Sometimes we are interested to find out if two approaches have the same effect. For instance we may like to find out the degree of agreement of two radiologists using a new technique. In such case we use the kappa statistic. In this technique we evaluate the real agreement in cells a and d (Table 26), when we eliminate agreement that happened by chance. Thus the initial apparent agreement of 72% is normalized to only 36%, when normalized for the agreement that occurs by chance. An agreement between 0 and 20% (κ between 0.0 and 0.2) is considered poor, between 20 to 40% fair, 40 to 60% good, 60 to 80% very good and over 80% excellent. The agreement found between the two radiologists will be considered fair.

NOMINAL OUTCOMES OVER TIME – SURVIVAL ANALYSIS

So far we have dealt with patients with a nominal outcome at a point in time – for example alive or dead after so much time. Often we are involved with studies where the outcome (nominal) is assessed, not at one particular

Table 26 Agreement in interpretation of radiographs between two radiologists

		Radiologist A		
		Positive	*Negative*	
Radiologist B	Positive	320	80	400
	Negative	90	110	200
		410	190	600

$$\kappa = \frac{\text{proportion of observed agreement} - \text{proportion of agreement by chance}}{1 - \text{proportion of agreement by chance}}$$

$$\kappa = \frac{(a + d)/N - (a_e + d_e)/N}{1 - (a_e + d_e)/N}$$

where a and d represent the values for a and d expected by chance and calculated as:

$a_e = (a + c) \times (a + b)/N = 400 \times 410/600 = 273$
$d_e = (d + c) \times (d + b)/N = 190 \times 200/600 = 63$

$$\kappa = \frac{0.72 - 0.56}{1 - 0.56} = 0.36$$

point in time but instead is followed over time. By the end of the study, the subject will belong to one of three categories: dead, lost to follow-up, or still alive (censored). Since everyone was not necessarily started in the study at the same time, it may be difficult to evaluate the data properly. For instance, a patient who registered only in the last two years of the study and is alive at the conclusion of the study does not allow us to draw any conclusions about whether he is expected to survive for a given longer period of time.

There are two techniques commonly used to show the probability of survival (*p*) at a given point in time; the **actuarial approach** and that of **Kaplan–Meier**. In both, the probability of death (q) within a period of time will equal the number of subjects that died in that period (D) over the number of subjects at risk at the beginning of the period. This, in turn, equals the number of subjects available at the beginning of the period minus the sum of subjects lost to follow up and these censored, all divided by 2. If *p* is the survival rate then q is equal to 1 – *p*. The major difference between these two statistical approaches is that the time interval is regular (i.e. every year) in actuarial analysis, while it varies in Kaplan–Meier. In Kaplan–Meier a similar analysis takes place for the time interval among two sequential events (deaths). Table 27 shows the status of subjects at the end of study, the time interval between registration and final event and their analysis for actuarial or Kaplan–Meier analysis. Figures 16, 17, 18 schematically depict the data as actuarial, Kaplan–Meier, and both.

Table 27a   Status of the subjects that participated, at the end of the study

Subject	Length of total (months)	
1	73	censored
2	53	lost
3	63	died
4	27	died
5	17	lost
6	44	died
7	92	died
8	61	died
9	20	died
10	105	censored

Table 27b   Status of the subjects participating in the study, at different time intervals

Number of years (cumulative)	Number at risk	Died	Lost/censored	Survival (interval)	Survival
0–1	10	0	0	1.00	1.00
1–2	10	1	1	0.89	0.89
2–3	8	1	0	0.87	0.77
3–4	7	1	0	0.86	0.66
4–5	6	0	1	1.00	0.66
5–6	5	2	0	0.60	0.40
6–7	3	0	1	1.00	0.40
7–8	2	1	0	0.50	0.20
8–9	1	0	1	1.00	0.20

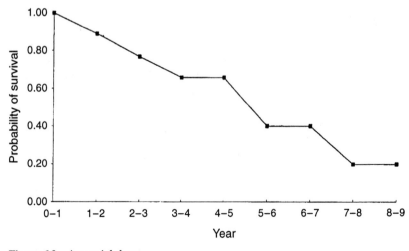

Figure 16   Actuarial data

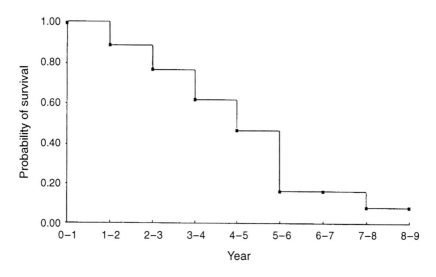

Figure 17   Kaplan–Meier data

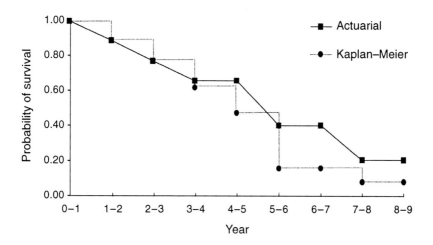

Figure 18   Actuarial and Kaplan–Meier data

If two different survival curves are compared (i.e. survival with therapy A vs. B), the difference between the probabilities of survival p among the two groups in a given time interval is similar to that shown for comparison of groups proportions, that is to say:

$$Z = \frac{P_1 - P_2}{SEM} = \frac{P_1 - P_2}{\sqrt{SE(P_1)^2 + SE(P_2)^2}}$$

where $SE(p) = P\sqrt{(1-P)/R}$

R = subjects at risk at the beginning of the time inteval.

Let us assume we would like to evaluate the probability of survival in the fourth year of treatment among patients with a given malignancy treated with either chemotherapy or radiation therapy. Let us say that the probability of survival is 0.2 for the chemotherapy group, which had 20 patients at risk at the beginning of that year while the radiation therapy group had a probability of 0.4 and 36 patients at risk.

Then $SEM_{pchemo} = 0.2\sqrt{(1-0.2)/20} = 0.04$

and the $SEM_{prad} = 0.4 = \sqrt{(1-0.4)/36} = 0.0516$

thus $Z = \dfrac{0.2 - 0.4}{\sqrt{0.04^2 + 0.0516^2}} = -3.06,$

$p < 0.002,$

thus one will conclude that radiationtherapy has a higher rate of survival than chemotherapy in the fourth year of treatment. Another way for comparing survival curves is that of the **logrank test**. Do not panic, it is a misnomer! There are no logarithms or ranks. In this test one tabulates the time that an event took place from smallest to largest. Then the number of patients at risk, as well as occurrences (i.e. failures or deaths), is determined for each time. Also, the number of expected occurrences for every group is identified by multiplying the total occurrences by the proportion of a given group represented in the patients at risk (that is patients at risk in the group under consideration over the total number of patients at risk for both groups). In Table 28, where two different treatments are compared for therapy in a malignant disease, the sum of observed occurrences (O) and expected occurences (E) is calculated. The expected occurrences are identified from the total number of occurrences at a given time relative to the proportion of patients at risk in a given group, as already suggested. Then one uses an approximate χ^2 where:

$$\chi^2 = \frac{(O_1 - E_1)^2}{E_1} + \frac{(O_2 - E_2)^2}{E_2}$$

Where O_1 and O_2 are the observed events and E_1 and E_2 the expected

Table 28 Hazard function analysis

Month of occurrence (positive, death)	Patients at risk			Occurrences			Expected occurrences		
	Treatment A	Treatment B	Total	Treatment A	Treatment B	Total	Treatment A	Treatment B	Total
2	22	25	47	1	2	3	1.40	1.60	3
5	21	23	44	0	2	2	0.95	1.05	2
7	20	20	40	2	1	2	1.00	1.00	2
10	18	17	35	2	0	1	0.51	0.49	1
11	17	17	34	0	2	2	1.00	1.00	2
13	16	15	31	0	1	1	0.52	0.48	1
16	16	12	28	0	2	2	1.14	0.86	2
19	15	10	25	1	1	1	0.60	0.40	1
22	14	9	23	0	1	2	1.22	0.78	2
24	13	7	20	0	1	1	0.65	0.35	1
Total				4	13	17	8.99	8.01	17

$$\chi^2 = \frac{(O_1 - E_1)^2}{E_1} + \frac{(O_2 - E_2)^2}{E_2}$$

$$\chi^2 = \frac{(4 - 8.99)^2}{8.99} + \frac{(13 - 8.01)^2}{8.01} = 5.88, \, p < 0.02$$

It suggests that, indeed, treatment A resulted in less occurences (i.e. deaths) in general over the 24 months of observation events in groups 1 and 2, respectively. Then we consult Appendix XI for χ^2 distribution for one degree of freedom. A similar test is the **Mantel–Haenzel χ^2 test**, that combines a series of 2×2 tables at different times during the survival analysis and allows for comparison of the survival curves.

One last method to deal with survival analysis is that of **hazard function**. Hazard function is the probability that a subject dies at a given time interval (say 6 years). The probability $H = d/(\Sigma f + \Sigma c)$, where d is the number of deaths, Σf is the sum of time in study of subjects that died, and Σc is the sum of all censored times. Based on the data of Table 28, in 8 years there were 6 deaths, that happened in 20, 27, 44, 61, 63 and 92 months (sum = 307 months). The sum of cenored time is $105 + 73 = 178$ months. Thus $H = 6/(307 + 178) = 0.0124$, which suggests that about 0.0124 patients die per month. Of interest, is that the reciprocal of H is equal to mean survival. In our example $1/0.0124 = 80.64$ which is consistent with a mean survival (κ) of 81 months. One may even obtain a reasonable approximation of the 95% confidence interval of survival if we calculate the $SEM(\kappa) = \sqrt{\kappa^2/d}$, or in our example $\sqrt{81^2/5} = 33.07$. Therefore one can be 95% confident that survival is $81 \pm (1.96)(33.07)$ or between 16.18 and 145.82 months.

Let us return once more to the hazard function. If several factors operate to result in death we may assume that each factor participates so that $(h_1 = h_0\, e^{(\beta 1 \times 1 + \beta 2 \times 2 + \ldots \beta x)}$, where h_1 and h_0 are the hazard factors at the time and when all x variables were 0. β_1, β_2 are regression coefficient slopes calculated for each factor separately. This is the **Cox[1] regression, or proportional hazards model**.

TAKE HOME MESSAGES

- χ^2 is the preferred test for groups having outcome in a nominal scale.
- Use **Fisher exact test** if one of the cells has a value of less than 5 or the total number of subjects is less than 20.
- **Relative risk** could be used in **prospective data**, and **odds ratio** in **retrospective** data.
- Proportions can be compared using the **z test**, if groups consist of more than 20 subjects each.
- For paired analysis (i.e. the effect of two treatments in the same subjects), one has to use the **McNemar** statistic.
- If one wishes to evaluate the degree of similarities (i.e. agreement) in paired analysis, then one should perform a **kappa** analysis.
- **Actuarial analysis**, or **Kaplan–Meier** analysis, should be used for **survival curves**.

---

[1]Proposed by the British statistician Sir David Cox (1972)

- **Log rank** and **hazard model** can also be used for **comparison of survival curves**.

QUESTIONS

1. Malnutrition is considered to be a major factor in determining the outcome of patients admitted to the medical intensive care unit. One hundred consecutive patients were divided into two groups based on their serum albumin: the hypoalbuminemics (serum albumin less than 3 g/dl) and the normoalbuminemics (serum albumin higher than 3 g/dl). Out of 52 patients with low albumin, 28 expired during this admission. By contrast, only 6 out of the remaining 48 died. Is there indeed a significant difference between the two groups?
2. What is the odds ratio describing mortality between the hypoalbuminemic and the normoalbuminemic? Is the difference statistically significant?
3. How do you deal with patients lost to follow up when you construct a survival curve? What about patients alive at the end of the study who have not been followed up for the entire time interval (i.e. patients alive in 3 years – when the study ended – and who have not been followed for 5 years in this 5-year survival study)?
4. Two skin tests are evaluated for evidence of normal immunity in 200 normal subjects.

		Test A		
		Positive	Negative	
Test B	Positive	123	14	137
	Negative	20	43	63
		143	57	200

Are the two tests different?
5. In the question 4 above, what is the agreement of the two tests?

CHAPTER 8

Put it all together – how to do a study and how to read the literature

Biology, and for that matter all science, advances by utilizing two selective methods: observation and experimentation. Observations, such as the relationship of occupation to pulmonary diseases, smoking to cancer, streptococcal infection to glomerulonephritis or endocarditis, are among the many examples of the significance of **observational** (often epidemiological) studies that have advanced our understanding of medicine. Interventions, on the other hand, are performed to alter physiology or pathophysiology and may allow us conclusions relative to the mechanism involved or potential treatment of diseases. (experimental studies) Table 29.

Observational studies can be further subdivided into those dealing with description of events but lacking control groups (case studies), and those comparing observations in the group under investigation against those in a control group (controlled studies). Case studies also differ in that they describe events in an unplanned fashion and their significance stems from the fact that one may identify a relationship. For example, the finding by Goodpasture of the coexistence of two rare events, bleeding from respiratory tract and bleeding from the urinary system, raised the possibility that the two may share some property. It turned out that the antigenic similarity of pulmonary and glomerular basement membranes is indeed the common denominator accounting for the so-called Goodpasture syndrome.

Table 29 Study types

Types of Studies
A. Observational

1. Non-controlled studies	2. Controlled studies
Case studies	(a) Case–control (retrospective)
	(b) Cross-sectional
	(c) Cohort studies (prospective)

B. Experimental

In control studies we compare data from the experimental group to that of the control group. This can be done in a retrospective way by cross-over techniques or as prospective studies. For instance, the finding of increased incidence of myocardial infarction in autopsies of smokers compared to age- and sex-matched controls is an example of a retrospective (case–control) study. This issue can also be addressed in a prospective study where two populations (smokers and non-smokers) are followed for many years, and the occurrence of interest (myocardial infarction) is observed. The Framingham study represents such a prospective study. Prospective studies are superior to retrospective ones in that the groups and the occurrence of interest are identified in advance, which eliminates potential bias. As an example of bias in retrospective analysis one may argue that the autopsy study in our example had included only certain socioeconomic classes that frequent the hospital where the autopsies were performed, or that there existed other, difficult to separate, confounding factors. The obvious downside of the prospective studies is that they take the time dictated by the length of observation, and are expensive because you have to have personnel to follow patients for the long term.

Cross-over studies have the advantage of not being retrospective but of short duration. They involve the evaluation of a property on two groups. For instance, in an effort to answer the same question we asked before, we may evaluate the EKGs for evidence of previous myocardial infarction in the two groups we select prospectively. There are obviously some advantages to such studies, but they lack the property of long-term follow-up.

In any event, a logical scheme is that information from case studies or other reports make one formulate a hypothesis. Observational studies serve to strengthen this hypothesis and occasionally to advance to a theory. The obvious next step is to test this hypothesis (theory) by moving to an interventional (experimental) study. For example, the finding that patients eating low-protein diets show slower progress of renal failure, is an observational study that evokes the hypothesis that high protein consumption may lead to progression of renal failure. Like all observational studies, it has the potential of leading to erroneous conclusions. For example, those patients who follow a low- protein diet may also be the more compliant patients who also follow other instructions (antihypertensive therapy, phosphate binders). Thus, the results obtained may not be directly attributable to the effects of protein consumption. To answer that, a control study can be performed in which two different groups are matched with regard to their age, sex, weight, renal function and renal disease, and are randomly given diets with different protein contents. A method of assessing adherence to the prescribed diet can be done by determining N_2 kinetics or obtaining diet histories. If such a

Table 30 Evaluation

Evaluation of study methods
1. Sensitivity, specificity, predictive value
2. Accuracy
3. Precision

---

study design results in the same conclusion then the role of protein in progression of renal disease is much more convincingly established. Note, however, that experimental studies cannot always be performed. For instance, in our previous example examining the association of smoking to myocardial infarction, it would be necessary to randomly assign subjects to become smokers and non-smokers in order to eliminate factors related to differences in personality or genetic background. This is, of course, unethical and thus such a study cannot be performed (in this case the evidence is strong enough that such a study is not needed!).

In both observational and experimental studies one has to clearly identify one's goals, including the number of groups, number of subjects, and methods to be used. Also, one has to clearly identify how the samples can be reworked so as to afford the least possible loss. It is not enough to just select the first 20 people you encounter. For example, suppose one wishes to evaluate whether the prevalence of systemic lupus erythematous has increased. If a random number of people are recruited in a large department store, a higher prevalence will be found since the store is frequented mostly by women, and lupus occurs predominantly in females. For the same reason, one will conclude, erroneously regarding the trend in alcohol consumption if your random group is selected at a race course or at a convent. Random sampling implies that every person of the group under consideration has an equal chance of being selected.

Another significant issue to be addressed before a study is begun is the number of subjects needed for each group. This was dealt with in detail in Chapter 3. To review briefly, one has to decide what difference in absolute value or proportion will be acceptable, what level of significance (α) and power ($1 - \beta$) will be allowed and what is the variation (standard deviation) usually found for this determination.

The tests used to detect the property should be evaluated with regard to their sensitivity, specificity and predictive value of a positive and negative test (see Chapter 3), and also with regard to accuracy and precision of methods (Table 30).

The statistical techniques used can be identified by evaluating whether the data are continuous, ordinal or nominal, as we have previously discussed in detail (Chapter 1). The specific calculations that will be needed have been provided in great detail in Chapters 4–7.

Table 31   Evaluation

Evaluation of Studies

A. Specific questions
   1. Relevance

B. Methodology
   1. Sampling
      (a) Survey
      (b) Groups
      (c) Number of subjects

   2. Techniques
      (a) Accurate
      (b) Precise
      (c) Ethical

   3. Statistical evaluation

The final issue is with regard to the results and conclusions. Even if sample selection, number and methodology are appropriate, one has to carefully evaluate the results before a valid conclusion is acceptable. For example, an average decrease of 2 mmHg in mean BP may be unacceptable for any antihypertensive medication, even if it reaches statistical significance. Similarly, the conclusions should be carefully evaluated for their true meaning. Again, if an antihypertensive medication promotes itself by showing that it decreased 10-year mortality rate by 50%, it may simply mean that the mortality has decreased from 1% to 0.5%. Instead, it brings up another question: Is it worth subjecting somebody to life-long treatment with many possible complications, including worsening quality of life, for such an apparently trivial advantage?

In short, whether one contemplates performing a study or is about to review a study performed by somebody else, one has to ensure that appropriate care has been taken in sampling, method selection and interpretation of the results (Table 31). If the study is defective in any of them, this detracts from its validity and its conclusion and, in an extreme case, may invalidate it completely. I am sure nobody would want to put forth the effort, personnel, and funding only to obtain a worthless, unpublishable, or even misleading study. This is the reason that all studies should be carefully evaluated **before** they are actually performed.

CONCLUSION

More recently a more formal approach has been developed to deal with the practical application of statistics on everyday practice. This method has been **named evidence-based medicine**. Its major features have already been dealt with in some detail in Chapters 2 and 4. In the remaining text I would like to recapitulate the highlights of this fashionable and powerful technique. It applies existing literature to help with two type of questions: (a) how given information may help to establish diagnosis in a given patient? (b) is it appropriate to treat a patient with a given treatment? To deal with either question one has to search the literature for the best existing evidence, that is, articles that have the characteristics described in detail in the first part of this chapter. More specifically:

(a) How given information may help me to establish diagnosis in a given patient?

In this case one has to establish if the test has a good discriminatory function, and then apply the discriminatory effect to improve the certainty of a diagnosis in a given patient. From the sensitivity and specificity of a test (or finding) one may find the likelihood ratio of a positive result, LR+, (sensitivity / (1– specificity)) and the likelihood of a negative result, LR – ((1 – sensitivity)/specificity). It follows that the higher the LR+, or the lower the LR–, the more the test is discriminatory. Even better, if the ratio of LR+/LR– is more than 50, one may consider this test as good. The next step is to multiply the LR+ by the odds that the patient has a disease and derive a new odds ratio that includes the information from the test. Remember that odds = probability/(1 – probability), and probability = (1 + odds)/odds. Thus probability can be readily translated to odds and vice versa. For example, if the probability of diabetic nephropathy is 60% in a given patient, and the LR+ for the presence of diabetic retinopathy is 15, then the new odds ratio will be equal to the LR+ (15) times the old odds ratio (0.6/0.4 = 1.5), i.e. 22.5, which translates back to probability (22.5/23.5 = 0.957). Thus, now one feels quite comfortable that the patient has diabetic nephropathy.

(b) Is it appropriate to treat a patient with a given treatment?

If a treatment is being considered, one has to identify the relative and the absolute reduction ratio (that is the amount of morbidity or mortality that is expected to decrease as a result of the treatment, based on the literature). Furthermore, one may extrapolate the number of patients needed to treat with such regimen so as to get at least one individual to avoid morbidity or death (NNT). Actually NNT = 1/ARR, where ARR is the absolute reduction rate. One will have to identify if the gains in morbidity and mortality due to the treatment are worth the effort , when compared against complications due to treatment, quality of life, and cost. Thus, a more appropriate decision could be made, often tailored to the specific needs of a patient.

Answers

Chapter 1

1. The outcome (i.e. cardiac output) is measured in a continuous scale (l/min). The dependent variables are either a control group or a group receiving an experimental drug (nominal, bivariable, two groups). If you go to Table 1, you find out, that the appropriate method to use is the Student *t*-test. If you plan to use the same subjects sequentially (to act as both control and experimental) one shall use the paired Student *t*-test. To avoid bias you may elect to randomise the subjects so as to prevent a constant sequence. Thus, in some, you evaluate first their cardiac output during baseline (control) conditions, and then you determine it following treatment with the experimental drug. In others, you first determine the cardiac output while receiving the experimental medication and then you determine the control cardiac output after they stop the drug (return to baseline).

    Alternatively, you may elect to randomly divide a group of subjects into control (subjects who will receive placebo or nothing) and experimental (those who will receive the experimental drug). You then determine the cardiac output in all subjects. The two groups in this case are unmatched and thus the Student *t*-test will be used.

    If the results appear not to follow a normal distribution, you then have to use non-parametric methods. For that, the Wilcoxon sign rank is the appropriate test if you plan to use a matched (paired) protocol, that is to say, if the same subjects will be used sequentially, both as control as well as experimental. If you plan to use two separate groups, then the Mann–Whitney U test is indicated (Table 1).

2. If two drugs will be evaluated, then you will have to deal with three groups: control, drug A, drug B. Since you deal with more than two groups, the appropriate selection is Repeated measures analysis of variance, if you use all three procedures in the same subjects (paired),

and a one way analysis of variance, if you plan to use three separate groups. If the data appear skewed, then the Friedman χ^2 test is indicated for the matched experiments, and the Kruskal–Wallis test for the unmatched ones.

3. In this case both the independent variable (24-hour urine creatinine), and the dependent variable (mid-arm circumference) are continuous (mg and cm, respectively). The appropriate method is linear regression.

4. In this question both the independent variable (type A) and the dependent variable (groups) are nominal. The correct method is then the χ^2.

Chapter 2

1a. As normal range we consider a range that includes 95% of the data. In a normal distribution this usually is equal to mean ± 2 standard deviations. In the present question, this is equal to $42 \pm (2 \times 2.5)$, or a range of hematocrits between 37 and 42.

b. A hematocrit of 39 is well within the normal limits as shown above.

c. The 95% confidence interval for the mean of a group is about equal to mean $\pm 2 \times$ SEM. As it was shown in Chapter 2, SEM = SD/$\sqrt{n}$. In the case under consideration, SEM = $2.5/\sqrt{25} = 0.5$.

Therefore the 95% confidence interval should be equal to $41 \pm 2 \times 0.5$, thus a range between 41 and 43 is where the mean of a group of 25 with normal hematocrits is expected. The fact that this group has a mean of 39 makes it different than normal. Note that while 39 is normal for a given individual, it is quite low if it represents the mean of a group.

2a. Let us consider a normal distribution with a point that allows 80% of the data to be higher, and 20% lower, than it. In such case one side will contain a 0.2 of the total (total = 1). If we check in Appendix I, we find that such a point is represented by a $z = 0.8$. This means that this point will be 0.8 standard deviations away from the mean. The mean is 64, implying that 50% of students had a score higher than 64. The remaining 30 will be within $0.8 \times$ SD = $0.8 \times 8 = 6.4$ or about 7 points less. The cut off should be placed at 57 to ensure a success rate of 80%.

b. 60 is 4 points less than 64. Given a standard deviation of 8, 60 is $4/8 = 0.5$ SD away from the mean. If we look at Appendix I, we find that a $z = 0.5$ indicates a one-side value of 0.3. This suggests, that if 60 is used as the cut off, 30% will have a score lower than that, and therefore will result in a success rate of 70%.

3. The answer is 5% (initial) +5% of the remaining 95% (about 4%) for a total of 9%.

4.   PROBABILITY

	Prior	Conditional (Granular casts)	Intermittent	Conditional ($\uparrow$ urine Na^+)	Posterior
PR	0.5	0.01	0.013	0.02	< 0.001
ATN	0.5	0.75	0.987	0.95	0.999

As shown in Chapter 2, for Bayes analysis, the intermittent probability for ATN is equal to

$$\frac{0.5 \times 0.75}{(0.5 \times 0.75) + (0.5 \times 0.01)} \quad \text{and the final one}$$

$$\frac{0.987 \times 0.95}{(0.987 \times 0.95) + (0.013 \times 0.02)}$$

Thus the diagnosis of ATN has a probability in excess of 99% based on the presentation.

5. If we solve the equation for Poisson distribution we find:
$P(0) = 0.01$
$P(1) = 0.03$
$P(2) = 0.08$
$P(3) = 0.14$
$P(4) = 0.18$
$P(5) = 0.18$
$P(6) = 0.15$
$P(7) = 0.10$
$P(8) = 0.07$
$P(9) = 0.04$
$P(10) = 0.02$
$P(11) = 0.01$
$P(12) = 0.003$
The probability of anything between 0 and 8 admissions in one day can be calculated by adding $P(0) + P(1)..... + P(8)$ and is about 0.94. This, between 0 and 9 admissions, is about 0.98. Therefore, the chief of nephrology should request between 8 and 9 beds to be sure he will accommodate his patients in about 95% of the time. The probability he may have 10 admissions in one day is low (about 2%). Two admissions in one day has a chance of about 8%.

6. The range that gives a 95% confidence in proportions is about equal to mean proportion $\pm 2SEM$. $SEM = \sqrt{p(1-p / n)} (n = \sqrt{20 \times 80/20}$ = 8.94. Thus, the expected range for a group of 20 is $20 \pm 2 \times 8.94$ or between 2.11 and 37.89%. This, in 20 subjects, suggests complications can happen from as little as almost no case to as high as 8. Ten is higher than this range and confirms your fear that there are problems with this kind of surgery in your Institution.

Chapter 3

1. If the prevalence of RVH is 2% this means that 200 patients out of a total number of 10 000 hypertensives have RVH. Since the sensitivity is 95%, then 190 of the 200 RVH patients will give a positive test. Since the specificity is 90%, this suggests that 8820 out of the 9800 hypertensives without RVH will have a negative Captopril test.

	+ Captopril	− Captopril
RVH	190	10
Other HTN	980	8820
Total	1170	8830

Therefore, only 190/1170 (16%) of the patients with a positive Captopril test will have RVH if this test is used as a screening test for RVH in the entire hypertensive population.

2. If the Captopril test is used as a screening test in a hypertensive population with a high prevalence (65%) then:

	+ Captopril	− Captopril
RVH	62	3
Other	3.5	31.5
Total	65.5	34.5

Thus, in this case, 62/65.5 (95%) of the Captopril positive test will indeed have RVH.

3. Since you do not want to miss a real effect, you will keep your α level at the highest acceptable level (thus you will not decrease it to less than 0.05). Similarly, you do not like to make the demonstration of a difference more difficult by increasing the power. The correct answer is neither (D).

4. In this case, we like to be strict and accept the existence of a difference only if we are thoroughly convinced. As a result, it is logical to tighten both α (to less than 0.05), and increase power to higher than 0.80 The correct answer is C.

5. As previously discussed, the number of subjects to participate in each group is:
$N = k* \sigma^2/\Delta^2$. The value of k can be found in Table 9 (Chapter 3). This is:

α	Power	k
0.05	0.80	7.849
0.01	0.90	14.879
0.05	0.95	12.995

By applying the appropriate values the answers are: (a) about 7 subjects per group, (b) about 13 subjects per group, and (c) about 3 subjects per group.

Chapter 4

1. To evaluate whether the difference among the two groups of nephrotic patients are different (and thus whether one treatment is indeed superior to the other one) we have to find the t value and then evaluate in Appendix II whether this t suggests a real difference. Since $t = \Delta / \sqrt{(s^2/n_1) + (s^2/n_2)}$, you then apply the following values to the formula:
    Δ = the difference of the two means i.e. 1 g
    s = standard deviation = 2
    n_1, n_2 = 25 subjects for each group.
    If you solve for t you find $t = 1.77$, consistent with no significant difference.
2. If we consider that now n_1, $n_2 = 100$, then $t = 3.54$, a difference highly statistically significant, $p < 0.001$.
3. The only difference from the situation above, is that $\Delta = 2$. As a result $t = 3.54$ that gives a $p < 0.001$, and suggest a difference that is highly statistically significant.
4. In this case, $t = 2.12$, which for a degree of freedom of 6 ($n_1 + n_2 - 2 = 6$) is not statistically significant.
5. We calculate the sum of squares (SS), then divide them by the degrees of freedom (DF) and calculate the mean of sum of squares or variance (MS) and find their ratio (F).

	SS	DF	MS	F
Between groups	516.7	2	258.33	30.7
Within groups	202	24	8.42	

By examining F in Appendix III, we find that $p < 0.001$, suggesting that the groups are unlikely to come from the same population. This implies that significant differences exist between the groups. We then evaluate the different pairs of groups.

	Δ	Bonferoni		Student–Newman–Keuls	
		t	$p < 0.05$	q	$p < 0.05$
Groups A vs B	10	7.31	Yes	10.34	Yes
Groups B vs C	8.33	6.09	Yes	8.62	Yes
Groups A vs C	1.67	1.22	No	1.72	No

Chapter 5

1a. R of 0.7 for 16 patients is consistent with a high degree of statistical significance, $p < 0.001$ (see Appendix VII).
 b. No. It is r^2 (not r) that allows for an understanding of the proportion of data that reflects the extent that the independent variable is controlled by the dependent one. In this case:
    $r^2 = 0.7^2 = 0.49$. This indicates that 49% of the values of creatinine were predicted from changes in body weight.

c. No. A good linear regression does not necessarily suggest a cause and effect relation. For instance, both may be controlled by another third factor.

2. In the case of 10 people, the same r will have different significance ($p < 0.05$ instead of $p < 0.001$ found before – see Appendix VII). However, r^2 will remain 0.49, so that again the linear regression will explain 49% of the data.

3. The correct answer is C, as r^2 indicates the percentage that the independent variable is predicted from the dependent one.

4. Any relation with $r = 0.3$ has a $r^2 = 0.09$. This implies that the regression explains only 9% of the values of the independent variable. Thus, although statistically significant, the relationship is of little physiologic relevance.

5. The lack of additional strength when the two independent variables are consider together, most likely suggest that they depend upon each other. Indeed, body weight is dependent, to a great extent, on height.

Chapter 6

1. If we use a non-parametric method (Kruskall–Wallis) we find H = 17.4, again suggestive of some highly statistical significant difference ($p < 0.001$).The direct comparison of the groups will be:

	Student–Newman–Keuls			Dunn		
	Difference of ranks	q	$p < 0.05$	Difference of ranks	q	$p < 0.05$
Groups A vs B	133.5	5.61	Yes	14.83	3.977	Yes
Groups B vs C	103.5	6.46	Yes	11.50	3.083	Yes
Groups A vs C	30.0	1.87	No	3.33	0.894	No

2. In this case we have to use the Friedman test (or repeated measures ANOVA of ranks). The $\chi^2 = 8.07$ which for df = 2 gives a $p < 0.025$. The direct comparisons of the groups will be:

	Student–Newman–Keuls			Dunn	
	Difference of ranks	q	$p < 0.05$	Difference of ranks	$p < 0.05$
Groups A vs C	10.5	3.32	Yes	1.05	Yes
Groups A vs B	7.5	3.35	Yes	0.75	Yes
Groups B vs C	3.0	1.34	No	0.30	Yes

3. We shall use the Mann–Whitney sum rank test. We find a T = 45.5 for n (small), and n (large) = 9. This is consistent with a highly significant difference ($p < 0.01$).

4. In this case we use the Wilcoxon sign rank test. We find T+ = 0, and T– = 28 for a $p < 0.05$.

5. The rank of the two instructors among the 10 medical students is as follows:

Student	Instructor 1	Instructor 3	d	d^2
1	2	3	1	1
2	6	9.5	3.5	12.25
3	6	6.5	0.5	0.25
4	9.5	6.5	3	9
5	2	3	1	1
6	2	1	1	1
7	6	3	3	9
8	6	6.5	0.5	0.25
9	6	6.5	0.5	0.25
10	9.5	9.5	0	0
				34

Thus $R_s = 1 - [(6 \times 34)/(10 \times 99)] = 0.79$, which is statistically significant, $p < 0.05$.

Chapter 7

1.

	Survived	Died	Total
	24	28	52
	42	6	48
Total	66	34	100

	Survived					Expired		
Observed	Expected	O – E	$(O-E)^2/E$	Observed	Expected	O – E	$(O-E)^2/E$
24	34.3	10.3	3.093	42	31.7	10.3	3.347
28	17.7	10.3	5.994	6	16.3	10.3	6.50

Thus $\chi^2 = 18.93$. If we use the short-cut formula we find a similar result (19.01). Both are consistent with a highly statistically significant difference ($p < 0.001$).

2. The odds ratio for mortality is $(42 \times 28)/(24 \times 6) = 8.17$. If we calculate the 95% confidence interval, using the formula provided in Chapter 7, we find that the ratio is between 2.94 and 22.55. This suggests that 1 (i.e. the possibility of mortality is equal between the two groups) is not a likely ratio, and we may conclude that mortality is statistically significantly different between the two groups. Similarly , the odds ratio for survival is the reverse, i.e. $(24 \times 6)/(42 \times 28) = 0.12$. In this case the 95% confidence interval is between 0.04 and 0.36. Again 1 is not part of this range, demonstrating that the two groups are statistically significantly different with regard to survival.

3. Patients that are still living at the end of the study but have not gone through the entire period set for the study, also have their data

incorporated in the analysis of survival. These observations are called censored, as we do not know how long these patients will stay alive. If we wish to calculate the mortality rate at a given interval (q_i), we have to divide the number of dead by the number of participants. As participants, we consider every person that started at this time interval, but we considered those lost to follow up or withdrawn from the the study before the end of the interval as one half: $q_i = d / [n_i - (0.5*w_i)$.

4. To answer this question we use the McNemar $\chi^2 = (b - c - 1)^2/(b + c)$ $= 49/34 = 1.44$. Thus the two tests are not significantly different.

5. To answer this question we will have to resort to the kappa analysis. The expected result by chance is equal to $137 \times 143/200 = 97.955$, while the d cell $= 63 \times 57/200 = 17.955$. Thus the agreement by chance is $(95.955 + 17.955)/200 = 0.57955$. The apparent agreement equals $(123 + 43)/200 = 0.83$. Then $\kappa = (0.83 - 0.57955)/(1 - 0.57955) = 0.6$. This suggests a very good agreement between the two tests.

Appendices

Critical values of z distribution

z	One-sided	Two-sided
0.00	50.00%	–
0.50	30.85%	61.70%
1.00	15.87%	31.74%
1.28	10.00%	20.00%
1.50	6.68%	13.36%
1.64	5.00%	10.00%
1.96	2.50%	5.00%
2.33	1.00%	2.00%
2.58	0.50%	1.00%
3.09	0.10%	0.20%

APPENDIX II

Distribution of *t* value

df	0.05	0.01	0.001
3	3.18	5.84	12.92
4	2.78	4.60	8.61
5	2.57	4.03	6.87
6	2.45	3.71	5.96
7	2.37	3.50	5.41
8	2.31	3.36	5.04
9	2.26	3.25	4.78
10	2.23	3.17	4.59
11	2.20	3.11	4.44
12	2.18	3.06	4.32
15	2.13	2.95	4.07
20	2.09	2.85	3.85
25	2.06	2.79	3.73
30	2.04	2.75	3.65
60	2.00	2.66	3.46
∞	1.96	2.58	3.29

APPENDIX III

Critical values of *F* distribution ($\alpha = 0.05$)

df Denominator	df, Numerator												
	1	2	3	4	5	6	7	8	9	10	15	20	100
4	7.71	6.94	6.59	6.39	6.26	6.16	6.09	6.04	6.00	5.96	5.88	5.80	5.63
5	6.61	5.79	5.41	5.19	5.05	4.95	4.88	4.82	4.77	4.74	4.62	4.86	4.37
6	5.99	5.14	4.76	4.53	4.39	4.28	4.21	4.15	4.10	4.06	3.94	3.87	3.67
7	5.59	4.74	4.35	4.12	3.97	3.87	3.79	3.73	3.68	3.64	3.51	3.44	3.23
8	5.32	4.46	4.07	3.84	3.69	3.58	3.50	3.44	3.39	3.35	3.22	3.15	2.93
9	5.12	4.26	3.86	3.63	3.48	3.37	3.29	3.23	3.18	3.14	3.01	2.94	2.71
10	4.96	4.10	3.71	3.48	3.33	3.22	3.14	3.07	3.02	2.98	2.85	2.77	2.54
11	4.84	3.98	3.59	3.36	3.20	3.10	3.01	2.95	2.90	2.85	2.73	2.65	2.40
12	4.75	3.89	3.49	3.26	3.11	3.00	2.91	2.85	2.80	2.75	2.62	2.54	2.29
15	4.54	3.68	3.29	3.06	2.90	2.79	2.71	2.64	2.59	2.54	2.40	2.33	2.07
20	4.35	3.49	3.10	2.87	2.71	2.60	2.51	2.45	2.39	2.35	2.20	2.12	1.84
30	4.17	3.32	2.92	2.69	2.53	2.42	2.33	2.27	2.21	2.17	2.01	1.93	1.62
60	4.00	3.15	2.76	2.53	2.37	2.25	2.17	2.10	2.04	1.99	1.84	1.75	1.39
∞	3.84	3.00	2.60	2.37	2.21	2.10	2.01	1.94	1.88	1.83	1.67	1.07	1.00

APPENDIX IV

Critical values of the q distributions (Tukey)
$\alpha = 0.05$

	2	3	4	5	6	7	8	9	10
1	17.97	28.98	32.82	37.08	40.41	43.12	45.40	47.36	49.07
2	6.09	8.33	9.80	10.88	11.71	12.44	13.03	13.54	13.99
3	4.50	5.91	6.62	7.50	8.04	8.48	8.85	9.18	9.46
4	3.93	5.04	5.76	6.29	6.71	7.05	7.35	7.70	7.83
5	3.64	4.60	5.22	5.67	6.03	6.33	6.58	6.80	7.00
6	3.46	4.34	4.90	5.31	5.63	5.90	6.12	6.32	6.49
7	3.34	4.17	4.68	5.08	5.36	5.61	5.82	6.00	6.16
8	3.26	4.04	4.53	4.89	5.17	5.40	5.60	5.77	5.92
9	3.20	3.95	4.42	4.76	5.02	5.24	5.43	5.60	5.74
10	3.15	3.88	4.33	4.65	4.91	5.12	5.31	5.47	5.60
11	3.11	3.82	4.26	4.57	4.82	5.03	5.20	5.35	5.48
12	3.08	3.77	4.20	4.51	4.75	4.95	5.12	5.27	5.40
15	3.01	3.67	4.08	4.37	4.60	4.78	4.94	5.08	5.20
20	2.95	3.58	3.96	4.23	4.45	4.62	4.77	4.90	5.00
30	2.89	3.49	3.85	4.10	4.30	4.46	4.60	4.72	4.82
60	2.83	3.40	3.74	3.98	4.16	4.31	4.44	4.55	4.65
∞	2.77	3.31	3.63	3.86	4.03	4.17	4.29	4.39	4.47

APPENDIX V

Critical Values for q (Student–Newman–Keuls)
$\alpha = 0.05$

	2	3	4	5	6	7	8	9	10
1	17.97	26.98	32.82	37.08	40.41	43.12	45.40	47.36	49.07
2	6.09	8.33	9.80	10.88	11.74	12.44	13.03	13.54	13.99
3	4.50	5.91	6.83	7.50	8.04	8.48	8.85	9.18	9.46
4	3.93	5.04	5.76	6.29	6.71	7.05	7.35	7.60	7.83
5	3.64	4.60	5.22	5.67	6.03	6.33	6.58	6.80	7.00
6	3.46	4.34	4.90	5.31	5.63	5.90	6.12	6.32	6.49
7	3.34	4.17	4.68	5.06	5.36	5.61	5.82	6.00	6.16
8	3.26	4.04	4.53	4.89	5.17	5.40	5.60	5.77	5.92
9	3.20	3.95	4.42	4.76	5.02	5.24	5.43	5.60	5.74
10	3.15	3.88	4.33	4.65	4.91	5.12	5.31	5.46	5.60
11	3.11	3.82	4.26	4.57	4.82	5.03	5.20	5.35	5.49
12	3.08	3.77	4.20	4.51	4.75	4.95	5.12	5.27	5.40
15	3.01	3.67	4.08	4.37	4.60	4.78	4.94	5.08	5.20
20	2.95	3.58	3.96	4.23	4.65	4.62	4.77	4.90	5.01
30	2.89	3.49	3.85	4.10	4.30	4.46	4.60	4.72	4.82
60	2.83	3.40	3.74	3.97	4.16	4.31	4.44	4.56	4.64
∞	2.77	3.31	3.63	3.88	4.03	4.17	4.29	4.39	4.47

APPENDIX VI

Critical values of a q statistics (Dunn)

K	a = 0.05	0.01	0.001
2	1.96	2.58	3.29
3	2.39	2.94	3.59
4	2.64	3.14	3.77
5	2.81	3.29	3.89
6	2.94	3.40	3.99
7	3.04	3.49	4.07
8	3.12	3.57	4.13
9	3.20	3.64	4.19
10	3.26	3.69	4.24
11	3.32	3.74	4.29
12	3.37	3.79	4.33
15	3.49	3.90	4.43
20	3.65	4.04	4.55
25	3.77	4.15	4.65

APPENDIX VII

Critical values of correlation coefficient, r

df	0.05	0.01	0.001
4	0.81	0.92	0.94
5	0.75	0.88	0.91
6	0.71	0.83	0.87
7	0.67	0.80	0.84
8	0.63	0.77	0.81
9	0.60	0.74	0.78
10	0.58	0.71	0.75
11	0.55	0.68	0.72
12	0.53	0.66	0.70
15	0.48	0.61	0.65
20	0.42	0.54	0.58
30	0.35	0.45	0.48
50	0.27	0.35	0.38

APPENDIX VIII

Critical values for Wilcoxon signed rank test (two-sided p value)

N	0.05	0.01	0.001
6	1	–	–
7	2	–	–
8	4	0	–
9	6	2	–
10	8	3	–
11	11	5	0
12	14	7	1
13	17	10	2
14	21	13	4
15	25	16	6
16	30	19	8
17	35	23	11
18	40	28	14
19	46	32	18
20	52	37	21
21	59	43	25
22	66	49	30
23	73	55	35
24	81	61	40
25	90	68	45
30	137	109	78
35	195	160	120
40	264	221	172
45	344	292	232
50	434	373	304

APPENDIX IX

Critical values of Mann–Whitney U statistics
$p < 0.05$

N_S	\multicolumn{12}{c}{N_L}
	4	5	6	7	8	9	10	12	14	16	18	20
2	–	10	12	14	15	17	19	22	25	29	32	36
3	12	14	16	19	21	23	26	31	35	40	45	49
4	15	18	21	24	27	30	33	39	45	50	56	62
5		21	25	29	32	36	39	47	54	61	68	75
6			29	34	38	42	46	55	63	71	80	88
7				38	43	48	53	63	72	82	91	101
8					49	54	60	70	81	92	103	113
9						60	66	78	90	102	114	126
10							73	86	99	112	124	138

APPENDIX X

Critical values for Spearman rank correlation coefficient, R_s

n	0.05	0.01	0.001
5	1.00	–	–
6	0.89	1.00	–
7	0.79	0.93	1.00
8	0.74	0.88	0.98
9	0.70	0.83	0.93
10	0.65	0.79	0.90
11	0.62	0.76	0.87
12	0.59	0.73	0.85
15	0.52	0.65	0.78
20	0.45	0.57	0.70
30	0.36	0.47	0.58
50	0.28	0.36	0.46

APPENDIX XI

Critical values of the Chi-square distribution
Probability (α)

df	0.05	0.025	0.01	0.005	0.001
1	3.841	5.024	6.635	7.879	10.828
2	5.991	7.378	9.210	10.597	13.816
3	7.815	9.348	11.345	12.838	16.266
4	9.488	11.143	13.277	14.860	18.467
5	11.070	12.833	15.086	16.750	20.515
6	12.592	14.449	16.812	18.548	22.458
7	14.067	16.013	18.475	20.278	24.322
8	15.507	17.535	20.090	21.955	26.124
9	16.919	19.023	21.666	23.589	27.877
10	18.307	20.483	23.209	25.188	29.588

Index